# Rad Histopathology

# Volume II

Author

## George W. Casarett, Ph.D.

Department of Radiation Biology and Biophysics
University of Rochester School of Medicine and Dentistry
Rochester, New York

This book is based on work performed under contract with the U. S. Department of Energy at the University of Rochester, Department of Radiation Biology and Biophysics.

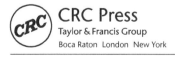

## CRC Press
Taylor & Francis Group
Boca Raton London New York

CRC Press is an imprint of the
Taylor & Francis Group, an **informa** business

CRC Press
Taylor & Francis Group
6000 Broken Sound Parkway NW, Suite 300
Boca Raton, FL 33487-2742

Reissued 2019 by CRC Press

A Library of Congress record exists under LC control number:

Publisher's Note
The publisher has gone to great lengths to ensure the quality of this reprint but points out that some imperfections in the original copies may be apparent.

Disclaimer
The publisher has made every effort to trace copyright holders and welcomes correspondence from those they have been unable to contact.

ISBN 13: 978-0-367-25518-3 (hbk)
ISBN 13: 978-0-367-25521-3 (pbk)
ISBN 13: 978-0-429-28822-7 (ebk)

Visit the Taylor & Francis Web site at http://www.taylorandfrancis.com and the
CRC Press Web site at http://www.crcpress.com

# PREFACE

Radiation histopathology may be defined here broadly as that branch of radiation biology which is concerned with the microscopic study of organized tissue and organ changes caused in vivo by radiation directly and/or indirectly. This book is concerned only with the effects of ionizing radiations on normal tissues and organs as observed by means of light microscopy.

Radiohistopathologic effects represent the consequences of cellular radiobiologic effects and constitute the bridge between cellular radiobiologic effects and gross pathologic and clinicopathologic consequences in the sequences of pathogenetic mechanisms of these gross effects and consequences. Although some biophysical and cellular radiobiologic background is provided, this is neither a cellular radiobiologic nor a clinical radiation pathology book, and is not intended to be a comprehensive treatise of the many and complex interdisciplinary facets of either of these fields. Nor is this book intended to be either an atlas, manual, or comprehensive reference source for radiation histopathology, but rather a treatment of this subject in pathogenetic terms with illustration of the principal features.

This book describes and illustrates the histopathology of ionizing radiations and discusses the pathogeneses of the major somatic degenerative, nontumorous, nonteratogenic effects of ionizing radiations. From the practical point of view, the principal thrust of the book is directed at those changes capable of developing into functional and/or structural impairments or lesions that may cause significant detriment in body systems and adversely affect health. The main focus of the book is the attempt to express radiohistopathologic observations in terms of the cellular dynamics of tissues and organs and to consider radiation histopathology in the general context of tissue response to injury rather than merely the special result of a specific type of injury or agent. As such, the treatment of the subject in this book is primarily concerned with general sequences, pathogeneses, and mechanisms, rather than with great detail and anecdotal material.

By means of reasonably broad classifications and generalizations, this book represents and consistently applies interpretations, theories, concepts, and schemes of relative radiosensitivity and of direct and indirect mechanisms of radiation damage of cells, tissues, organs, and systems in vivo which appear to be highly compatible with the experimental and clinical evidence and which permit reasonable prediction of radiopathologic damage. Permanent, progressive, and delayed radiation effects are considered as well as acute effects. The additivity of these radiation effects with other changes occurring with time or increasing age and the influence of this additivity on the time of appearance and degree of pathologic expression of the radiation injury are also stressed.

Most of the information on which these concepts and interpretations of pathogenetic sequences and mechanisms are based has come from extensive experimentation, with a lesser amount from occasional well-designed extensive studies of human organs and consideration of the aggregate of great numbers of more anecdotal human case reports. Disagreement with some of the author's interpretations, concepts, or criteria is expected in such an interdisciplinary, multilevel field of investigation as that of radiobiology in which there are still so many large gaps in knowledge. The gap between basic cellular radiobiology and clinical radiopathology is still very large. For purposes of study of pathogenetic sequences and mechanisms, there is more valuable radiohistopathologic information, and illustration, for some organs, which have been studied intensively for this purpose, than for other organs. For this reason, certain organs and tissues have been given more or less consideration and illustration in this book.

The illustrative materials used in this book are largely those developed from the research of, and for graduate teaching by, the author in the field of radiation histopathology over the past thirty years. The literature listed as being cited specifically and/or as other sources omits of necessity many of the vast numbers of publications which have more or less bearing on the subject. The references and other sources include those articles and books used in the review of specific subject matter. It is from this diversity of selected background information that the text of this book has been derived.

The author hopes that this book will help the reader, whether a researcher or clinician, to understand better the translation of cellular effects of ionizing radiation into subsequent detriment in the body.

**George W. Casarett, Ph.D.**

# ACKNOWLEDGMENTS

The author wishes to express his gratitude to all of those people who have contributed to the experience on which this book is based: to research scientists in this field, past and present; to his collaborators in research over the past three decades; to the many graduate students, who have contributed much of the information used in the book; and to his technical associates who have contributed vitally to his research.

Many thanks are owing to Beverly Holloway for her excellent secretarial and editorial capability in the production of this manuscript.

Most of all, the author wishes to convey his deepest gratitude to his wife, Marion, and daughter, Vicki, for their many kinds of vital support and encouragement.

George W. Casarett

# THE AUTHOR

**George W. Casarett, PH.D.** is Professor of Radiation Biology and Biophysics, and of Radiology at the University of Rochester School of Medicine and Dentistry, Rochester, New York.

Dr. Casarett obtained his premedical education at the University of Toronto (1938-1941) and the University of Rochester (1943-1945). He undertook his Graduate studies at the University of Rochester where he earned his Ph.D. in Anatomy (Pathology) in 1952. Since 1943, Dr. Casarett has held numerous Research and Academic positions at the University of Rochester School of Medicine.

Dr. Casarett is currently Chairman of Scientific Committees #1 and #14 of the National Council on Radiation Protection and Measurements, of which he has been a Director. He is a recent past Chairman of the National Academy of Sciences Advisory Committee on Biological Effects of Ionizing Radiation.

Among his numerous past activities in national and international organizations, Dr. Casarett has been a member of the National Academy of Sciences Advisory Committees to the Federal Radiation Council and to the Atomic Bomb Casualty Commission, the National Cancer Institute Research Training Committee, and Committee #1 of the International Commission on Radiological Protection, and a consultant to the United Nations Scientific Committee on Effects of Atomic Radiation and the Nuclear Regulatory Commission. His membership and Fellowship in numerous scientific societies include memberships in the American Association of Pathologists, Radiation Research Society (former councillor and associate editor of journal), American Association of Anatomists, and Society for Experimental Biology and Medicine.

Dr. Casarett has authored over 200 papers on various aspects of radiation research. His major fields of research are in Radiation Pathology, Radiation Biology, Carcinogenesis, Gerontology, and Cancer Biology.

# DEDICATION

For Marion

# TABLE OF CONTENTS

## Volume I

# TABLE OF CONTENTS

## Volume II

Chapter 1

RESPIRATORY TRACT

## I. HISTOLOGY

The nasal passage (excepting the continuation of the skin in the vestibule), the larynx, the trachea, and the bronchi and their branches are lined by pseudostratified, ciliated, columnar epithelium containing numerous goblet cells and resting on a basement membrane which is located between the epithelium and the underlying layer of connective tissue with its mixed mucous glands. The nasopharynx is lined by ciliated columnar epithelium. These epithelia are composed of reverting postmitotic cells which are relatively radioresistant.

The primary bronchi branch into secondary bronchi, and these into bronchioles, then terminal bronchioles, respiratory bronchioles, alveolar ducts, alveolar sacs, and alveoli (Figure 1A). The mucous membrane of the bronchi is continuous with that of the trachea and is of the same type (Figure 1B). The pseudostratified ciliated columnar epithelium rests on a basement membrane separating it from the lamina propria. Small cuboidal cells are found on the basement membrane in the epithelium of the trachea, bronchi, and their branches, and are usually the cells which divide when required to replace the more specialized cells which are lost. The turnover time of bronchial epithelium is relatively long.

The functional unit of the lung consists of a respiratory bronchiole and the structures extending from it, the alveolar ducts, alveolar sacs, and alveoli. The ciliated columnar epithelium of the bronchial tree changes to low cuboidal epithelium in the respiratory bronchioles. The short respiratory bronchioles branch into variable numbers of alveolar ducts of varying length, which are long, tortuous, thin-walled, branching tubes which give rise to thin-walled alveolar sacs (outpouchings containing more than one alveolus) or alveoli (Figure 1A). The alveolar duct wall between the openings of the alveolar sacs contains collagenous and elastic fibers and smooth muscle cells. The alveolar walls contain close, highly anastomosing networks of capillaries, supported by a fine network of reticular fibers, and a small number of elastic fibers. The alveoli are lined by a thin, simple, low epithelium separated from the capillary endothelium by a thin basement membrane (Figure 1C). The free macrophages that are sometimes found in alveoli (alveolar phagocytes) are like macrophages found elsewhere in the body. They are derived mainly from hematogenous lymphocytes and monocytes; the name septal phagocytes has been given to cells in the septa that have been observed to assume the appearance and function of macrophages.

Normally, the blood capillary networks in the alveolar walls are separated from the air only by a thin membrane through which oxygen and carbon dioxide easily diffuse. The reserve functional capacity of the normal lung is large, so that at rest the human body requires the use of only a small fraction (about 1/20th) of the aerating surface. The epithelial lining of the respiratory structures of the lungs consists of reverting postmitotic cells, which are relatively resistant to the direct destructive actions of radiation.

## II. RADIATION HISTOPATHOLOGY

So-called radiation pneumonitis may be regarded as an inflammatory reaction in which there is first a phase that is predominantly exudative. This reaction may either

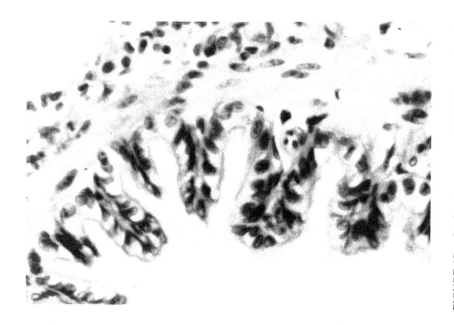

FIGURE 1B.    Section (approximately 800×) showing branch of bronchus.

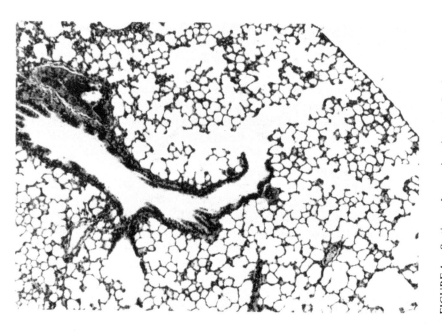

FIGURE 1.    Sections of normal rat lung. A. Section (approximately 100×) showing bronchial branch, terminal bronchiole, alveolar duct, alveolar sacs, and alveoli.

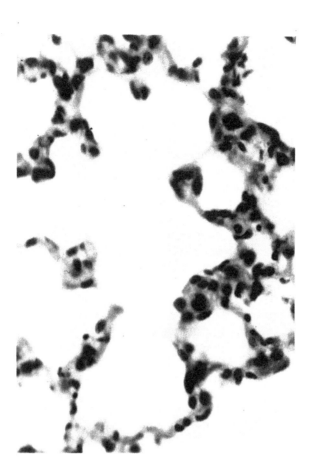

FIGURE 1C.    Section (approximately 800 ×) showing alveolar sac and alveoli. (H. and E. stains.)

resolve and leave little or no histopathologically detectable change, except perhaps for
subtle vascular changes, or it may progress to a chronic or delayed late phase with
chronic inflammation and fibrosis as the prominent features. On a clinicopathologic
basis, radiation pneumonitis cannot easily and at all times be sharply divided into acute
or exudative and chronic or fibrotic periods, since the earlier phase may merge subtly
or mix with the other, and complete or partial resolution may occur either early or
late in the overall process.

The inflammatory, degenerative, and fibrotic changes which radiation can cause in
tissues of various kinds are of special significance when they occur in the lung where
their presence interferes directly and early with vital and urgent functions. In the lungs,
as compared with more compact organs (those tightly encapsulated and relatively in-
active physically), hematogenous exudates more easily and rapidly enter critical functional space, the respiratory air space, in relatively large amounts, aided by the bellows-
like action of the lung. Therefore, the exudative aspects of the early or late periods of
radiation response easily and rapidly interfere with respiratory function by increasing
the barrier to the diffusion of gases between capillaries and alveoli, as well as by re-
ducing the available alveolar air space. Likewise, the dependence of the respiratory
function of the lung on a thin alveolar membrane and ready diffusion of gases allows
for rapid and easy interference with this function by a relatively small degree of increased cellularity or proliferative response as is involved in the inflammation and
fibrosis of radiation pneumonitis.

Because of the relative radioresistance of epithelial tissues of the lungs, the early and late consequences of irradiation of the lungs are due largely to vascular and connective tissue effects. Transient acute responses may be caused in the fine vasculature and connective tissue by relatively small or moderate doses (e.g., a few hundred to 1200 rads), and such responses increase in degree and duration with larger doses. The chronic and delayed effects in the lung are caused primarily by progressive vasculoconnective tissue changes with secondary effects on parenchymal cells. The complication of pulmonary infection may also play an important role in the development and persistence of the process in some cases.

Early histopathologic changes in the lung after irradiation include hyperemia and vascular congestion, edema of alveolar walls, lymphangectasia, exudation of proteinacous fluid from the blood into the alveolar spaces, leakage of red cells and diapadesis of hematogenous polymorphonuclear leukocytes into alveolar spaces, increases in phagocytic cells, increased mucus secretion by the bronchial epithelium, and some degenerative changes in small numbers of alveolar and bronchial epithelial cells, followed by rapid recovery of the latter changes.

The sequence of early changes (within two months after thoracic irradiation) in rat lungs after various single localized doses of X-rays (600 to 3600 rad) is illustrated in the following figures. Pulmonary congestion and edema, slight at two days, becomes more marked within a week. There is edema of alveolar walls, alveolar spaces, bronchial walls, vessel walls, and into pleural space, where fibrinous pleuritic membranes are formed on the outer lung surface (Figure 2). By two weeks after irradiation there has been virtually complete resolution of the alveolar edema, but alveolar walls are thickened at the expense of alveolar lumens, perhaps a result of infiltration of mononuclear cells, there are numerous alveolar phagocytes in some regions, and small arteries show degenerative and obstructive changes as well as persistent edema (Figure 3). There is also evidence of hyperplasia, disorganization, and some degenerative change in epithelium of bronchi, associated with the beginning of fibrosis in their submucosal tissue (Figures 4A and 4B). By one month after irradiation, there are foci of emphysema and areas of marked increase in mononuclear inflammatory cell infiltration in alveolar septal walls, and to a lesser extent in alveolar spaces associated with relatively dense fibrinous deposits in alveolar spaces (Figure 4C). Occasional fibroblasts or transitional forms between mononuclear cells and fibroblasts are present in alveolar septa or spaces (Figure 4D). By the second month after irradiation, the process of chronic inflammation and fibrosis is more active and extensive, depending on dose, both in alveolar walls and spaces and in pleuritic membranes (Figure 5).

Jennings and Arden[148], in their studies on rats, found that there was little significant difference in the changes in lungs subjected to single or fractionated exposures. Septal thickening was of about the same degree in animals given 3000 rads of thoracic irradiation fractionated at 600 rad per week for five weeks and those given 1000 rads followed in 50 days by 2000 rads, as compared with a single dose of 3000 rads. They cited one possible differential effect of fractionation, a response of the pulmonary blood vessels. At 60 days after irradiation, those animals given the dose fractionated for five weeks at 600 rads per week showed a more marked thickening of blood vessels than was seen in the other groups. Many of the smaller blood vessels in the lungs showed prominent subintimal hyalinization. At times, later than two months after irradiation, the changes in the alveolar septa appeared to be slowly progressive. At the end of a year there was marked generalized fibrosis in alveolar septa throughout the lung, with the alveolar walls being three to six times as thick as normal. The thickening was due chiefly to proliferation of fibrillar tissue. Reticulum fibers proliferated and condensed. The fibrosis appeared to be the result of the organization of the persistent fibrin-rich edema fluid seen in the alveolar septa soon after irradiation.

5

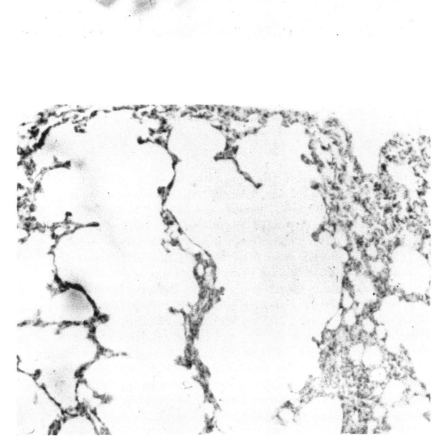

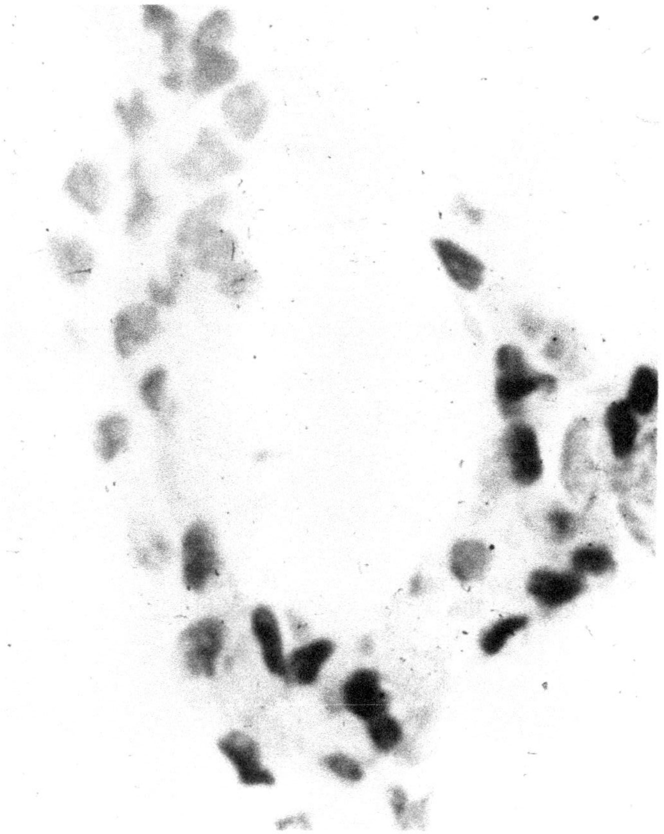

FIGURE 2B. Section (approximately 1,000×) after 1200R, showing edema of alveolar walls.

FIGURE 2. Sections of rat lungs 1 week after thoracic X-irradiation. A. Section (approximately 100×) after 600R, showing an area of edema and emphysema.

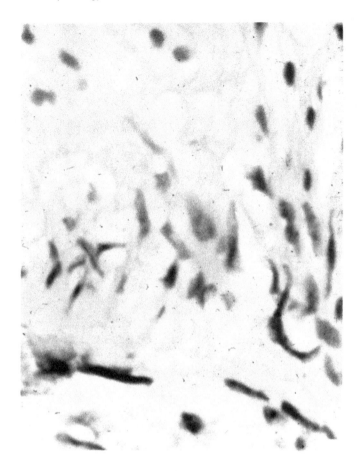

FIGURE 2C.   Section (approximately 1,000×) after 1200R, showing medial degeneration, edema, and the beginning of fibrosis in the wall of the
pulmonary artery.

Warren and Spencer[155] described the hyalin membrane in the alveoli in radiation
pneumonitis in human beings as a reliable diagnostic sign of radiation injury, whereas
others regard this change as nonspecific. Jennings and Arden[149] attempted to evaluate
and correlate dosage and time factors in the development of radiation pneumonitis in
human beings by reviewing autopsy records and slides of 173 cases of therapeutic irradiation to the thoracic region. The doses range from less than 500 to more than 6000
rads. Presence or absence of the following tissue changes was noted: edema, congestion, atelectasis, fibrin exudate in the alveoli, epithelial changes, fibrillar thickening
of alveolar septa, increased cellularity of alveolar septa, fibrosis of alveolar septa, and
proliferative changes in blood vessels. The incidence of edema, congestion, and atelectasis was not significantly different from that seen in nonirradiated lungs. The accumulation of fibrin-rich exudate within alveoli and the thickening of alveolar septa by
fibrillar material, cellular proliferation, or fibrous tissue were the two changes presumably caused by irradiation that were especially frequent in this study. The other
changes commonly attributed to radiation were not as constant. Little epithelial degeneration was observed.

The outpouring of alveolar edema fluid rich in fibrin, associated with the initial
congestion and edema, in the absence of cellular inflammatory changes, suggests that
injury to the fine vasculature plays a primary role in the development of this charac-

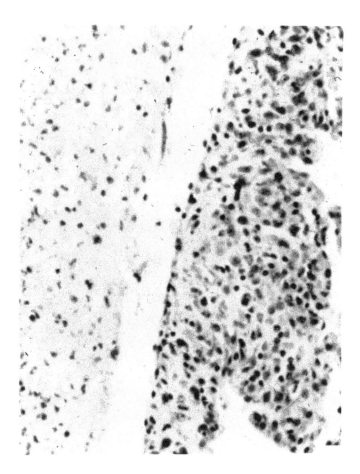

FIGURE 2D. Section (approximately 400×) after 600R, showing a fibrinous pleuritic membrane (left) which was adherent (but became detached in tissue processing) to the surface of the lung (right) and had formed from plasmatic transudation from the lung. The periphery of the lung shows thickening of alveolar walls with hematogenous mononuclear (chronic inflammatory) and connective tissue cells. (H. and E. Stains.) (From Kurohara, S. and Casarett. G. W., unpublished photomicrographs).

teristic picture of early radiation pneumonitis. The fibrin condenses at the alveolar walls to produce the so-called hyalin membrane. Jennings and Arden[149] found fibrin membranes in 41% of all irradiated human lungs in their study, most frequently and most prominently six months to two years after doses greater than 2000 rads. There seemed to be little difference in the appearance of the fibrin membranes in alveoli produced by different doses, regardless of the time of observation, for example, fibrin accumulations within three months after 1500 rads as compared with those nine years after 5000 rads.

In the development of fibrosis of alveolar walls, the appearance of fibrillar structures in the interstitial edema fluid is a fairly early change and, together with the fairly early infiltration and proliferation of histiocytes and the proliferation of reticulum, it contributes to increased thickening of the alveolar walls. At least some of the fibroblasts which can appear in the alveolar walls may have been developed from the histiocytes. In association with the accumulation of fibroblasts, there is a gradual fibrous thickening of the alveolar walls.

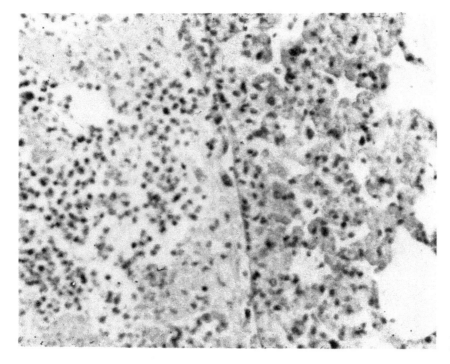

FIGURE 3B.   Section (approximately 400x) showing inflammatory cell infiltration and early fibrosis of the fibrinous pleuritic membrane (upper half of picture), and congestion and thickening of the pulmonary alveolar walls (lower half of picture).

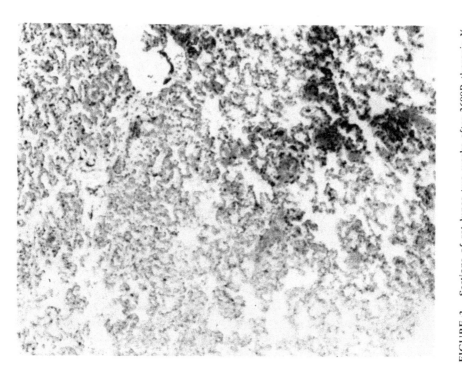

FIGURE 3.   Sections of rat lungs two weeks after 3600R thoracic X-irradiation. A. Section (approximately 100x) showing general thickening of alveolar walls at the expense of alveolar air space.

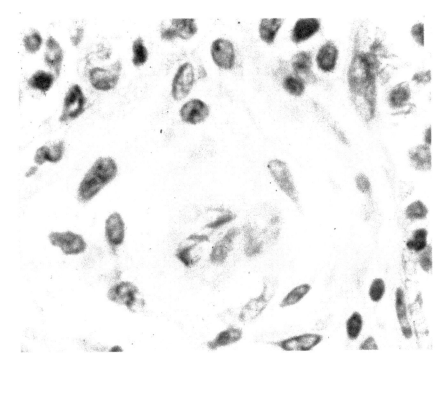

FIGURE 3D. Section (approximately 1000×) showing small artery with thickened, edematous, fibrotic wall, and obliteration of lumen. (H. and E. stains.) (From Kurohara, S. and Casarett. G. W., unpublished photomicrographs).

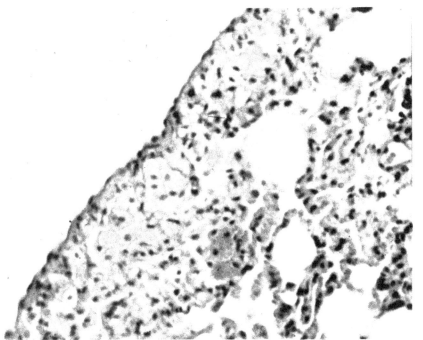

FIGURE 3C. Section (approximately 400×) showing numberous alveolar macrophages in area at periphery of lung.

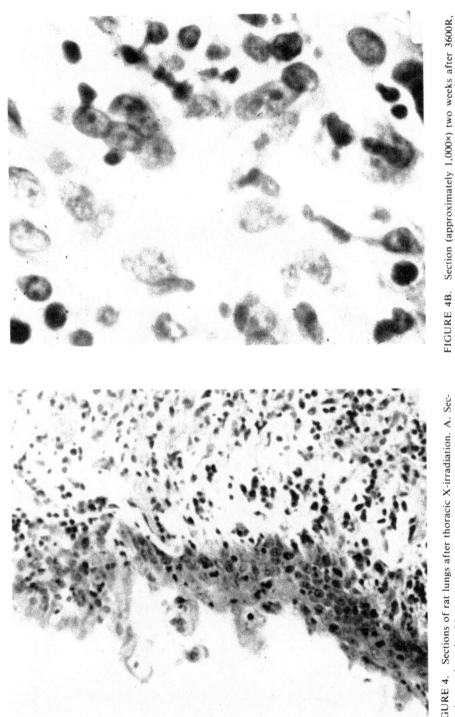

FIGURE 4B.    Section (approximately 1,000×) two weeks after 3600R, showing chronic inflammatory cells and some active fibroblasts in the submucosa of a bronchus.

FIGURE 4.    Sections of rat lungs after thoracic X-irradiation. A. Section (approximately 400 ×) two weeks after 3600R, showing disorganization, hyperplasia, degeneration, and chronic inflammation of the mucosa of a bronchus overlying an inflamed fibrosing submucosa.

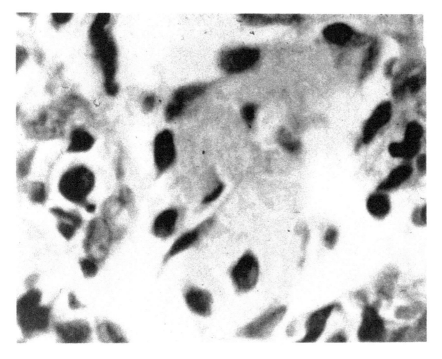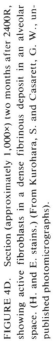

FIGURE 4D. Section (approximately 1,000×) two months after 2400R, showing active fibroblasts in a dense fibrinous deposit in an alveolar space. (H. and E. stains.) (From Kurohara, S. and Casarett, G. W., unpublished photomicrographs).

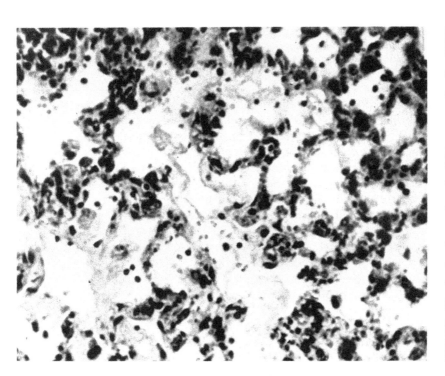

FIGURE 4C. Section (approximately 400×) one month after 2400R, showing marked mononuclear inflammatory cell infiltration in alveolar septal walls and to a lesser extent in alveolar spaces associated with relatively dense fibrinous deposits in alveolar spaces.

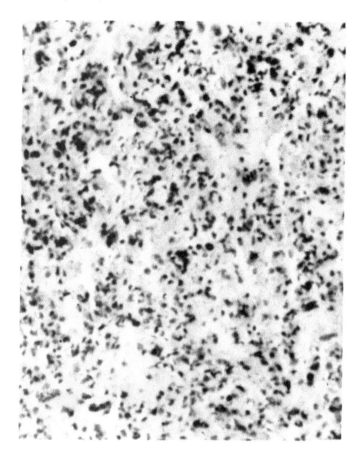

FIGURE 5.   Sections of rat lungs two months after 2400R thoracic X-irradiation. A. Section (approximately 200×) shows an area of chronic inflammation and early fibrosis with markedly diminished alveolar air space.

In their study of irradiated human lungs, Jennings and Arden[149] found that increased deposition of fibrillar connective tissue in alveolar septa was most frequent after radiation doses greater than 3000 rads and after postirradiation intervals longer than six months, although it did occur at shorter intervals or, in the case of smaller doses, at long intervals. There seemed to be either some time dependence associated with this change or little recovery from this change, in that the fibrillar thickening of alveolar walls 65 days after 4500 rads was similar to that present many years after a similar dose. The increased accumulation of histiocytes and fibroblasts in the alveolar walls was seen most frequently at dose levels between 2000 and 5000 rads, and the condition at six months was similar to that observed at two years after similar doses of radiation. Fibrosis of the alveolar walls (with dense fibrous tissue) could be found in a month or two in some cases after relatively large doses, but was fairly frequent at periods longer than six months after doses of 500 rads or greater.

On the basis of their experimental work on dogs, Fleming et al.[146] have associated the pathogenesis of radiation pneumonitis with defective lung plasminogen activation, which appears by the end of the first week after doses of 1500 to 2000 rads of $^{60}$Co gamma rays. They reasoned that with the lung's fibrinolytic system thus paralyzed, fibrin deposits persist and lead to hyalin membrane formation and ultimately to fibrosis of the lung.

13

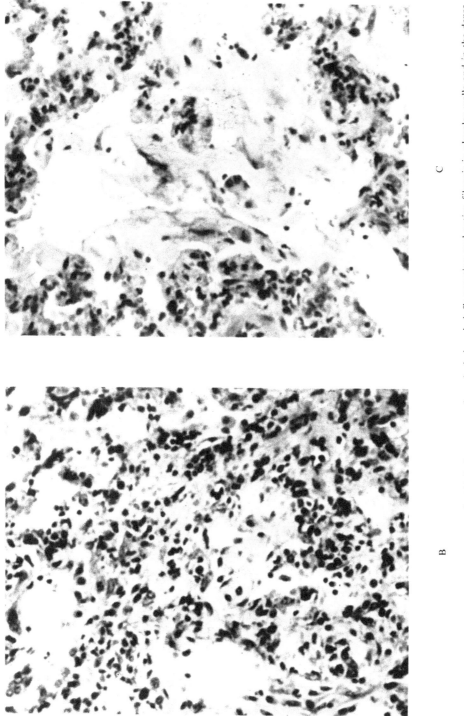

C

B

FIGURE 5B and 5C. Sections (approximately 400×) show areas of marked chronic inflammation and active fibrosis in alveolar walls and in the dense fibrinous deposits in alveolar spaces.

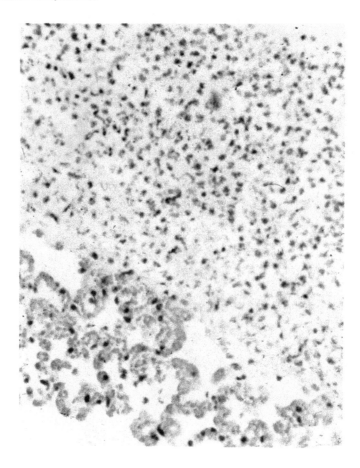

FIGURE 5D.   Section (approximately 200×) shows chronic inflammation and early fibrosis of a fibrinous pleuritic membrane attached to the
surface of the lung where the alveolar walls are congested, but otherwise
fairly normal. (H. and E. stains.) (From Kurohara, S. and Casarett, G.
W., unpublished photomicrographs).

If the acute phase of the reaction (acute radiation pneumonitis) is mild, it may sub-
side in a few weeks or months, leaving little or no evidence of the reaction, although
subtle vascular and connective tissue changes may persist. These persisting changes
may progress or be supplemented by other changes, so that long after irradiation they
may contribute to delayed fibrosis in lungs. If this occurs a very long time after irradiation, it may be so subtle as to be regarded merely as a premature development of
the changes seen frequently in old age. If the acute phase of the reaction is severe, the
lung changes soon become chronic and may persist or progress for months or years,
with excessive proliferation of connective tissue, mainly in the alveolar walls; hyalinization and thickening of blood vessel walls and reduction of the fine vasculature; and
the development of areas of atelectasis, emphysema, and fibrosis. The fibrosis may be
regarded as a process of repair of the radiation damage by secondary intention, but it
may also in some cases be a reparative response to secondary infection as well.

It should be reemphasized at this point that the time intervals implied here by such
terms as acute, chronic, or late relate to progressive phases in pathogenesis. As in
radiation reactions in other organs, acute types of pathologic change may occur not
only soon after irradiation, but months or years later as well. The term acute is used
here to indicate the initial reactions to radiation injury which occur soon after irradia-

tion, that is, early vascular damage, congestion, edema, early cellular infiltration of the alveolar walls, early fibroblastic formation and fibril formation, etc., as distinguished from later chronic conditions which persist or progress, such as alveolar fibrosis and arteriosclerosis.

In summary, in the reaction of lung to irradiation, a prime role is played by the damage and response of the fine vasculature (capillaries, arterioles and venules) and the connective tissue elements, which result in endothelial swelling and proliferation, thrombosis, congestion, increased permeability of vessels, edema and fibrinous exudation, chronic inflammatory cell infiltration, and fibroblastic activity. Resolution of the severe acute phase is accompanied by further fibrosis, vascular obstruction or obliteration, slight bronchial epithelial proliferation, sclerosis of connective tissue, and varying amounts of calcification. This process results in a loss of cilia, increased secretions, areas of atelectasis and compensatory emphysema, increased cellularity of the alveolar walls, congestion and edema, secondary infection, more fibrosis and atelectasis, and bronchiectasis. Pleural effusions and adhesions may also occur. Lung tissue affected with these progressive changes is increasingly liable to subsequent breakdown as a result of inherent progressive damage or of complications brought about by infections or other insults or stresses.

The doses of radiation required to cause marked acute histopathologic reactions are highly variable, although generally the doses are relatively large. Variations in the radiation dose rate and quality, volume of lung tissue irradiated, part of lung irradiated, as well as the size of the total dose, all may influence the development of the lesions. The reserve lung volume and capacity and the status of the lung (disease, aging change) before irradiation also contribute to the marked variability in time and degree of development of acute lesions. The difficulty in explaining the great variability of the reaction on the basis of these factors suggests that there are still other important factors to consider. Pulmonary infection may be an important one, and so may be the role played by damage to the lymphatic channels in certain parts of the thorax.

The degree or rate of progression of the residual vasculoconnective tissue changes depends largely on the size of the dose, the dose rate, and the degree and persistence of the acute reaction. Following the more severe persistent acute reactions, the lungs may continue to show combinations of acute and chronic types of histopathological changes, with a tendency toward predominance and progression of the chronic changes (parenchymal fibrosis) and a greater degree of progression of arteriolocapillary sclerosis, occlusion, and reduction.

In the experimental studies by Michaelson et al.[151] of dogs given single doses of 1000 kVp X-rays to the upper body (thorax, neck, and head) tachypnea at rest, with marked hyperventilation on exercise, was noted as early as seven months following a single dose of 1750 rads and nine months after a single dose of 1500 rads. Arterial blood oxygen saturation was reduced. Death occurred 10 months after the delivery of 1750 rads and 11 months after 1500 rads. With single doses below 1500 rads, evidence of respiraory difficulty did not become manifest until more than 12 months after irradiation. The postmortem findings of thickened alveolar walls, diffuse pulmonary fibrosis, and vascular thickening and occlusion correlated well with the development of progressively more severe arterial blood oxygen unsaturation and moderate hypercapnia. It appeared to the authors that in the earlier stages of this syndrome, alveolar capillary block played a primary role in the arterial unsaturation because of the absence of significant concomitant hypercapnea. This interpretation was further supported by the blood-gas analysis following exercise, which indicated arterial unsaturation in the presence of eucapnea or hypocapnea. It was thought that the later changes in which there was a moderate hypercapnea coupled with severe arterial oxygen unsaturation may

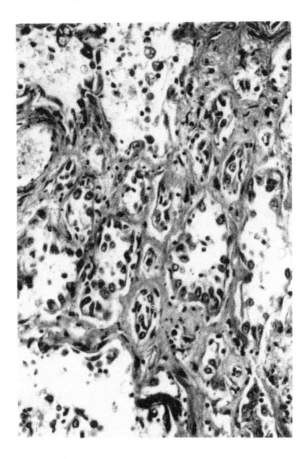

FIGURE 6.    Sections of dog lungs approximately a year after
1700R thoracic X-irradiation. A. Section (approximately 400×)
shows marked dense fibrotic thickening of alveolar walls and
fine vasculature, metaplasia of alveolar septal cells, and
chronic inflammatory cells and alveolar phagocytes in the alveoli.

well have represented a terminal degree of pulmonary fibrosis associated at least partly
with a defect in ventilatory distribution as well.

The chronic and delayed radiation damage in lung tissues, in the form of sclerosis
and reduction of the fine vasculature and increased parenchymal fibrosis (Figure 6),
even if not inherently progressive with passing time (as it may well be after substantial
damage), may be additive to similar changes occurring with passing time as the result
of the pathologic effects of various agents and of inherent aging processes. These combined changes constitute a progressive sclerotic deterioration of the lung parenchyma,
with a gradual reduction in the functional reserve capacity and in the tolerance to
additional infection, insult or stress, such that the delayed problems of pulmonary
fibrosis may become evident years after irradiation. When the initial irradiation effects
and residual damage are only very mild, the late uncomplicated picture may well be
described as premature aging of the lung.

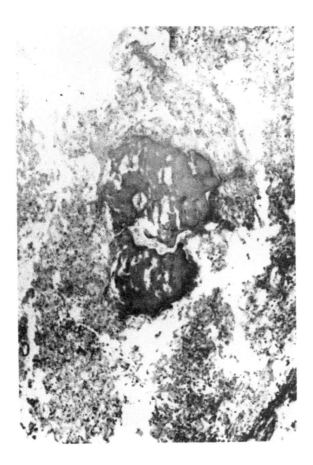

FIGURE 6B. Section (approximately 100×) shows bone-like formations in the fibrotic lung. (H. and E. stains.)

Chapter 2

# URINARY TRACT

## I. RENAL HISTOLOGY

The kidney is a compound tubular merocrine gland containing structures (glomeruli) in the course of its vasculature which filter waste substances from the blood, and tubules (proximal convoluted, collecting, loops of Henle, distal convoluted) which act on the glomerular filtrate (adding to, removing from, and concentrating) to produce concentrated urine. The kidney is composed of an outer cortex (Figure 1A), with its glomeruli and proximal and distal convoluted tubules and collecting tubules, and an inner medulla which contains some of the loops of Henle and the collecting tubules which lead to the pelvis and the openings of the ureters.

The blood vasculature of the kidney is abundant, and about one-fifth of the body's blood passes through the kidneys per min. Interlobar arteries arise as branches of the renal artery, pass between the pyramids of the kidney, and become arcuate arteries at the cortical-medullary junction. The interlobular arteries are branches of arcuate arteries and follow a radial course through the cortex. The interlobular arteries give off branches to the glomeruli (afferent arterioles) which, after breaking up into the glomerular capillary loops, reform as efferent arterioles which supply capillaries surrounding cortical tubules (Figures 1B and 1C). The interlobular arteries also give off some terminal branches to the renal capsule and subjacent cortex, and the efferent glomerular arterioles, in addition to supplying the blood vessels of the nearby cortical tubules, also give off branches (arteriolae rectae) to the medulla from efferent arterioles near the medulla. The tubules of both the cortex and the medulla are surrounded by capillary plexuses arising from the efferent arterioles of the glomeruli. It is probable that the convoluted tubules of each nephron are usually supplied with the blood that has just passed through the glomerulus of that nephron. Renal arterioles tend to be end arterioles, the only supply to the regions served.

The glomerulus (Figure 1D) is a lobulated spheroidal mass of looped and tangled capillaries interposed in the course of an arteriole and nearly completely enveloped by a double-walled glomerular capsule. The efferent arteriole is smaller than the afferent arteriole, and the points of entry and exit of these vessels are close together (vascular pole of the glomerulus). Near its entrance to the glomerulus, the media of the afferent arteriole has a modified structure in that the smooth muscle cells become large, pale, lacking in myofibrils, and epitheloid in appearance, and they contain variable numbers of granules. This myoepitheloid part (the juxtaglomerular apparatus) is closely associated anatomically with the macula densa of the ascending limb of Henle's loop (Figure 1D).

## II. RENAL RADIATION HISTOPATHOLOGY

The simple epithelium of the renal tubules and of the glomerular capsule are long-lived reverting postmitotic cells which rarely divide under normal conditions, but which can respond to certain strong stimuli or to a loss of cells by proliferating. Such cells are relatively resistant to the direct destructive actions of radiation. Parts of nephrons can be replaced by newly regenerated cells, but new nephrons are not formed. Consequently, there tends to be a loss of nephrons with increasing time as a result of injury or aging. The total nephron loss is partly compensated by the hypertrophy of other tubules and glomeruli.

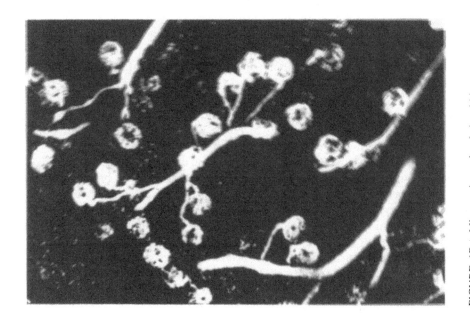

FIGURE 1B.    Microangiograph of dog kidney cortex (approximately 100×), showing afferent glomerular arterioles branching from interlobular arteries and entering glomeruli.

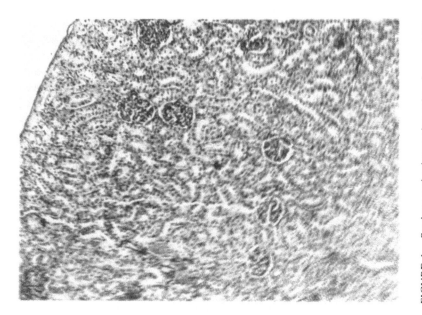

FIGURE 1.    Sections and microangiographs of normal kidneys. A. Section of rat kidney cortex (approximately 100×).

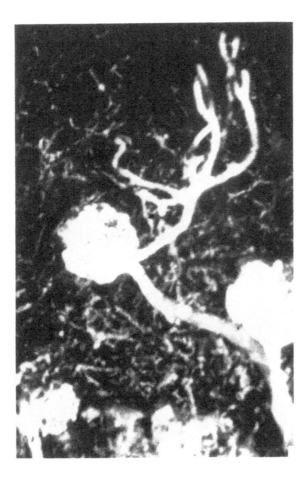

FIGURE 1C. Microangiograph of rat kidney cortex (approximately 400×), showing the afferent and efferent glomerular
arterioles of a glomerulus (center of picture), branches of the
efferent arteriole, and peritubular capillaries.

The precise mechanisms of the radiation induction of renal damage are not yet entirely clear, and much of the relationship between morphological alterations and functional changes has yet to be clarified. However, considerable progress has been made
toward these objectives.

The findings and opinions of the earlier experimental investigators concerning the
primary site of radiation injury in the kidney and the pathogenic sequences following
injury were greatly conflicting or controversial, and some of the controversy still remains. The earlier studies on irradiation of the kidneys of experimental animals, which
denied the existence of significant renal damage, largely involved short-term observation periods, and relatively little special attention was paid to vascular changes, especially in the finer vessels. Other earlier studies did reveal damage to the kidney, but
often the radiation dose could not be clearly defined at the time (especially before
1925).

It has now become largely accepted that the kidney is moderately susceptible in terms
of the relatively late effects of radiation, although the relative radiosensitivity of the
tissue components and precise sequence of direct and indirect mechanisms in the pathogenesis remain to be completely clarified and are still in some dispute.

At varying times after irradiation was administered under various conditions, differ-

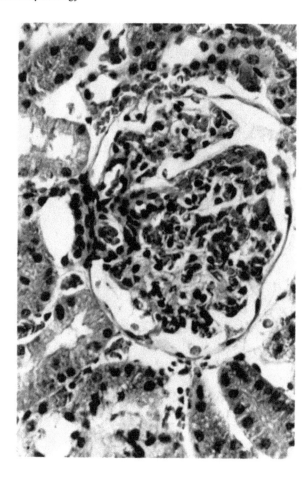

FIGURE 1D.    Section of dog kidney cortex (approximately 800×) showing a glomerulus (center of picture) with its afferent and efferent arterioles (within the glomerulus). (H. and E. stains.) (B and D from Maier, J. G. and Casarett, G. W., U.S. Atomic Energy Commission Report UR-626, 1963; C from Eddy, H. A. and Casarett, G. W., unpublished.)

ent proportions of the following general histopathologic changes, among others perhaps, have been noted in irradiated kidneys of experimental animals or of man: (1) degeneration, necrosis or atrophy of the tubular epithelium; increased interstitial connective tissue, thickening of basement membranes; (2) hyalinization of connective tissues; (3) replacement fibrosis of renal structures; (4) degeneration, necrosis, swelling or proliferation of endothelial cells; (5) vascular intimal thickening, endarteritis, medial degeneration, necrosis or thickening of blood vessel walls and narrowing of lumens; and (6) degeneration, necrosis, or atrophy and scarring of glomeruli. Also the association of hypertension and its consequences secondary to radiation-induced renal damage has become recognized.

Casarett[62,65,159] elucidated some sequences and mechanisms in the pathogenesis of radiation-induced renal disease in an histopathologic study of rats sacrificed at intervals after single intravenous injections of various dosages of polonium-210, a practically pure alpha emitter with negligible chemical significance in amounts used, which is excreted largely via the kidneys. Polonium retention studies indicated that the major portion of the continuous irradiation of the kidneys was completed in two or three

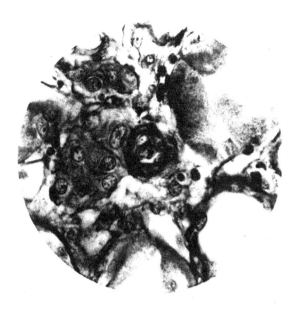

FIGURE 2. Sections of kidney cortex of rats showing obstructive changes in fine vasculature in the early stage of radiation-induced arteriolonephrosclerosis. A. Arteriole (center of picture) nearly completely occluded by endothelial proliferation; (approximately 400×).

months. Casarett distinguished the pathogenesis of the progressive renal damage as an arteriolonephrosclerotic process, distinct from the pathogenesis of other types of nephritis or nephrosis. The essenial histopathogenesis of arteriolonephrosclerosis (ANS) consists of:

1. Damage of endothelium and narrowing and/or occlusion of arteriolar (and capillary) lumens, at first by endothelial swelling and proliferation (later by fibrosis) (Figure 2);
2. Initiation of a progressive hypertensive process (increasing systolic pressure);
3. Degeneration and hypoplasia of cortical tubule cells secondary to persistent and progressive vascular damage from irradiation and hypertension, without regeneration of epithelium (Figure 3);
4. Progressive degeneration and sclerosis of vasculature (Figure 4), including glomeruli, with impairment of circulation (Figure 4);
5. Progressive loss of parenchymal epithelium (without regeneration) and progressive replacement fibrosis (Figure 5);
6. Reduction of the kidney to a sclerotic mass.

In the late stages of nephrosclerosis caused by irradiation, the sclerotic, contracted kidney is difficult to distinguish from the "secondarily contracted kidney" seen late in the processes of other types of nephritides.

Following the establishment of this arteriolonephrosclerotic mechanism of radiation damage of kidneys in polonium-treated rats by Casarett, this process was also demonstrated in experiments on dogs and rats irradiated with X-rays. These studies include one by Maier and Casarett[169] on dogs receiving unilateral or bilateral renal X-irradiation in single doses (500, 1000, or 2000 rads), which confirmed this pathogenesis for external irradiation. This pathogenesis was also confirmed by Wachholz and Casar-

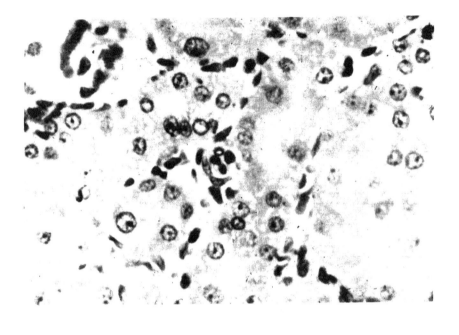

FIGURE 2C.   Arteriole (center of picture) occluded by swollen and degenerate endothelial cells; (approximately 800×).

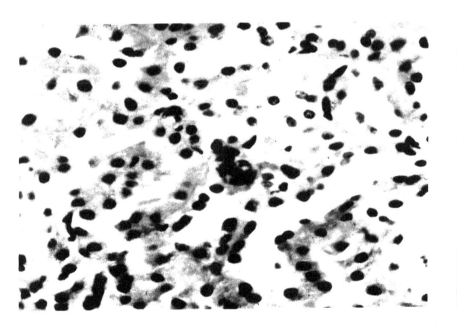

FIGURE 2B.   Arteriole (center of picture) occluded by endothelial cells and fibroblasts; (approximately 400×).

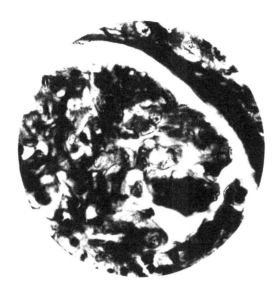

FIGURE 2D. Glomerulus showing endothelial occlusion of capillaries in many locations; (approximately 1,000×). (H. and E. stains.) (A and D from Casarett, G. W., *Radiat. Res. Suppl.*, 5, 246, 1964. With permission. B from Wachholz, B. W. and Casarett, G. W., unpublished; C from Rappaport, D. and Casarett, G. W., unpublished.)

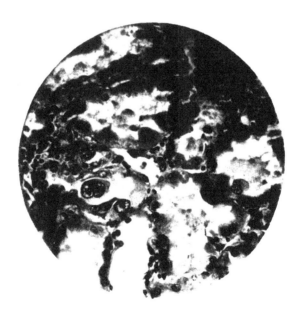

FIGURE 3A. Sections of kidney cortex of rats showing early degeneration and loss of epithelium of convoluted tubules secondary to vascular and circulatory impairment in radiation-induced arteriolonephrosclerosis. A. Epithelial cells of convoluted tubules show degeneration, necrosis (pyknosis, karyolysis, cytolysis), enlargement, and division anomalies; (approximately 400×). (A—D from Casarett, G. W., *Radiat. Res. Suppl.*, 5, 246, 1964. With permission.)

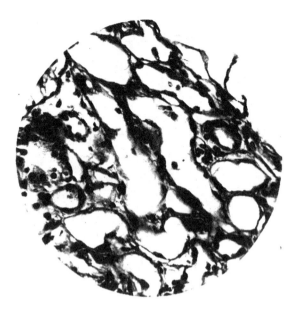

FIGURE 3B.   Marked loss of epithelium in convoluted tubules in regions of greatest vascular impairment; (approximately
400×).

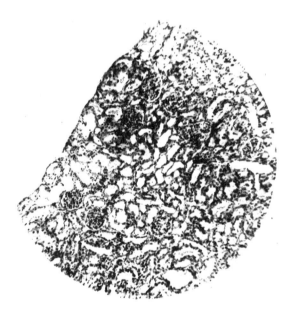

FIGURE 3C.   Section (approximately 100×) shows considerable early loss of epithelium from convoluted tubules, compared with the normal cortex (see D).

ett[177] in rats irradiated with X-rays (300, 500, or 1000 rads) to the kidneys only, the
whole body, or the whole body with kidneys shielded. All three modes of irradiation
caused similar dose-dependent degrees of hypertension. It was shown that the hypertension began to develop in association with the early and relatively subtle arteriolar
changes in the kidneys or the rest of the body, before considerable changes developed

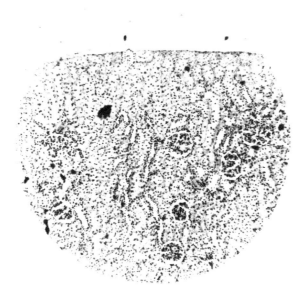

FIGURE 3D. Normal rat kidney cortex (approximately 100×). (H. and E. stains.) (From Casarett, G. W., *Radiat. Res. Suppl.*, 5, 246, 1964. With permission.)

in tubular epithelium. The progressive hypertension in turn contributed much to the degenerative changes in arterioles and other arteries especially in previously irradiated vessels, with the establishment of a vicious cycle between vascular damage and hypertension and consequent parenchymal loss and replacement fibrosis.

The bulk of evidence now favors the fine vasculature as the histologic site of damage of primary importance in the pathogenesis of radiation-induced nephrosclerosis (arteriolonephrosclerosis). The renal epithelium is relatively resistant to the direct destructive actions of radiation, but it may degenerate as the result of damage to the fine vasculature, and in doing so may cause regressive changes in vessels of various sizes. The larger blood vessels of the kidney may also be affected indirectly as a result of radiation changes in the small vessels and as a result of hypertension caused by renal radiation, all of which may indirectly cause degeneration of the tubular epithelium. The rate of this whole process tends to be slow after small doses and rapid after large doses, or after moderate doses given in schedules which are critical for eliciting persistent occlusive endothelial reactions in small vessels.

The early histopathologic changes in the kidney are similar to those seen in many other tissues after irradiation. There is early hyperemia and increased capillary permeability (as judged by dye injection) which results in interstitial edema (plasma exudate) which separates capillaries and tubules. Endothelial cells of the fine vasculature reveal degenerative and necrotic changes or swell and bulge into the lumen, and subsequently, as if in response to this damage, they regenerate and increase in number, sometimes excessively, and occlude the lumen. In some instances, especially after large or intensive doses that kill the endothelium and prevent regeneration, arterioles and capillaries show fissuring or thrombosis. The afferent glomerular arterioles are especially susceptible near the hilus of the glomerular tuft, but other arterioles and also some glomerular and tubular capillaries are also affected.

These occlusive changes in the fine blood vessels, possibly with functional vasoconstriction as well, result in impedence or obstruction of the circulation of the blood.

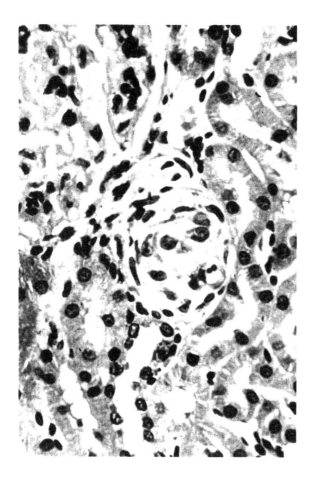

FIGURE 4.   Sections of kidney cortex showing later changes
in fine vasculature after X-irradiation. A. Section (approximately 800×) from rat after 1500R showing sclerotic thickening
and partial occlusion of arterioles (center of picture) with degeneration of associated glomerulus.

The kidney cortex becomes pale. Microangiographs can demonstrate the blocks in the
afferent glomerular arterioles dramatically in terms of the reduction in the number of
glomeruli filled with the radioopaque medium. Injection of a dye (e.g., Evans blue)
into the renal artery reveals reduced visibility of the dye in the pale, grossly observable
renal surface, as compared with nonirradiated kidneys. Autoradiography following
injection of radioactively labeled serum albumin is useful in demonstrating increased
permeability and plasmatic transudation through the endothelium of vasculature in
the kidney.

   These early changes in structure of the fine vasculature are subtle rather than con-
spicuous, and are variable in degree and spotty in distribution, such that the number
of vessels apparently altered in a given histologic tissue section of several microns of
thickness is relatively small and not representative of the number of small vessels actually altered, as can be seen better in microangiographs. The narrow lumens of small
blood vessels are relatively easily occluded and need only be occluded at one spot along
their course to impede blood circulation throughout their length. For these reasons,
microangiographs provide a more dramatic illustration of the substantial significance
of these early subtle changes than does histologic examination alone. Large renal blood

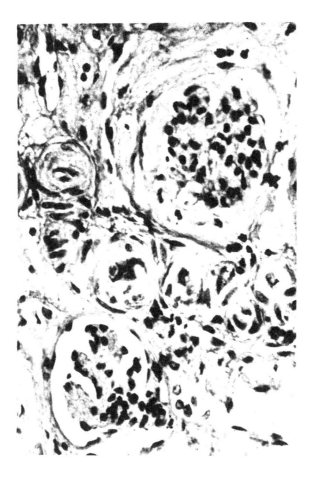

FIGURE 4B.    Section (approximately 800×) from dog six
months after 2000R, showing marked sclerotic thickening and
occlusion of arterioles, and degeneration and sclerosis of associated glomeruli in advanced arteriolonephrosclerosis.

vessels may be relatively unaffected initially, while the fine vasculature is affected.
Therefore an adequate examination of the kidney for vascular effects cannot be limited
to the more obvious vasculature. Furthermore, in view of the occlusion or obliteration
of the lumens of fine blood vessels, the identification of these vessels in examination
of the tissue sections should not rely heavily on the presence or identification of patent
lumens.

The spotty sites of plasma exudate outside of capillaries or in the subendothelial
regions of arterioles become sites of collagen deposition and of progressive degenerative and eventually fibrotic and sclerotic changes leading to increases in the amount,
density, and hyalinization of interstitial connective tissue, thickening of basement
membranes, fibrotic thickening of arteriolar walls with reduction of lumens, and degeneration and reduction of patent capillaries in the glomeruli and around the tubules.

Rapid mechanisms of occlusion of the small blood vessels with the production of
renal cortical ischemia include endothelial swelling and proliferation, and thrombosis.
Slower mechanisms involve the progressive degeneration and thickening of vessel walls
and narrowing of lumens without early involvement of the occlusive endothelial reactions or of thrombosis. Rapid or slow mechanisms that produce cortical ischemia, if
sufficiently marked and persistent, sooner or later cause progressive secondary degen-

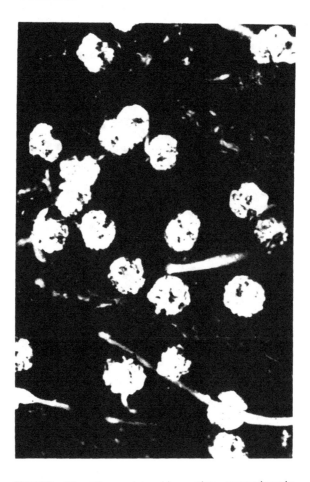

FIGURE 4C. Microangiographic section (approximately 200×) from normal nonirradiated dog kidney showing glomerular vascular filling for comparison with the following section.

eration of the dependent tubular epithelium and atrophy and reduction of cortical tubules.

The importance of the rapid mechanisms of vascular occlusion, involving persistent endothelial swelling and proliferation in small vessels in the early phases of arterionephrosclerosis, was demonstrated in the polonium experiments conducted by Casarett (1952 to 1964) on rats.[62-65] At comparable times after polonium injections, this nephrosclerotic process was much more rapid and severe at a dosage level of 10 μCi/kg body weight (about 2800 rad to the kidney in 200 days; only slightly more dose was added during the remainder of life) than at a dose level twice this size (20 μCi/kg). The 10 μCi/kg dosage injured the endothelium considerably, but still permitted these occlusive endothelial reactions. The higher dosage (20 μCi/kg) caused such great endothelial damage that such reactions were prevented, and the secondary degeneration and loss of tubular epithelium were much smaller at comparable time than that at the 10 μCi/kg level, despite the fact that the vessels were much more severely damaged and undergoing sclerosis of their walls. Similarly, later and smaller losses of epithelium were observed in rats given lower dosages (5 or 1 μCi/kg), which caused only minimal endothelial injury and little persistent endothelial reaction.

There is very little effort made at regeneration of tubular epithelium to replace the epithelium lost, as compared with the regeneration observed in other types of nephri-

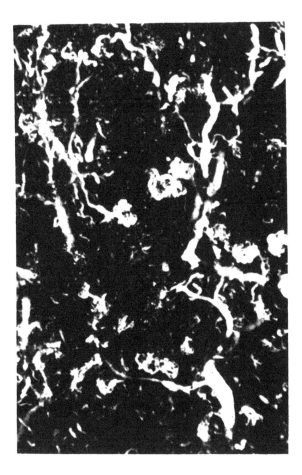

FIGURE 4D. Microangiographic section (approximately 100×) from dog six months after 1000R showing markedly decreased glomerular filling and dilatation, engorgement, and tortuosity of interlobular arteries and afferent arterioles. H. and E. stains.) (A from Rappaport, D. and Casarett, G. W., unpublished; B, C, and D from Maier, J. G. and Casarett, G. W., U.S. Atomic Energy Commission Report UR-626, 1963.)

tides which are not caused primarily by vascular and circulatory impairment. This would be expected on the basis of the persistence and progression of vascular changes causing the ischemia; successful regeneration would not be expected under such conditions if these conditions were the cause of the epithelial loss in the first place.

The cortical tubules, especially the convoluted tubules, seem to be more affected in the ANS process than the medullary tubules. The slowly progressive secondary degeneration and loss of tubular epithelium, without regeneration (due to poor vascular support), leads to denudation and atrophy of tubules, gradual collapse of the cortex, and gradual replacement of tubular and glomerular structures by connective tissue.

Aside from considerations of optimal critical doses and/or dose rates for persistent endothelial obstruction of arterioles, the rate of progression of the arterionephrosclerotic process after irradiation depends generally on the dose size (and dose rate). For example, by the end of six months the arterionephrosclerotic process in dogs has progressed to a marked degree after a single dose of 2000 rads, to a moderately marked degree after 1000 rads, and to a mild degree (with little tubular change as yet) after 500 rads.

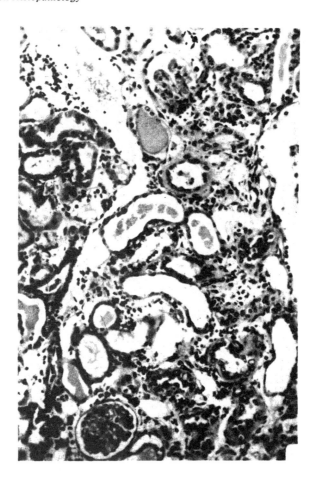

FIGURE 5.  Sections of kidney cortex showing progressive
tubular epithelial loss and replacement fibrosis in arteriolonephrosclerosis after X-irradiation. A. Section (approximately
400×) from a rat after 1000R, showing degeneration and necrosis of tubular epithelium, formation of tubular casts, and early
peritubular chronic inflammation and fibrosis.

The type of clinical symptomatology presented or type of renal disease represented
clinically at any particular time during the radiation-induced nephrosclerotic process
depends on the rate and stage of the nephrosclerotic process.

There may be stages mimicking so-called benign hypertension, in which renal damage as judged by renal function studies and urinalysis are minimal, chronic renal failure
with or without hypertension, chronic hypertension with or without renal failure, or
late malignant hypertension.[166] Death from radiation-induced nephrosclerosis may result from uremia, renal failure, malignant hypertension, cerebrovascular hemorrhage,
or congestive heart failure.

## III. URETERS AND BLADDER

The calyx-pelvis structures of the kidneys, which are expansions of the ureters, include the minor calyces, the double-walled cups fitting around the projecting pyramid
tips, the major calyces formed by several minor calyces, and the renal pelvis, into

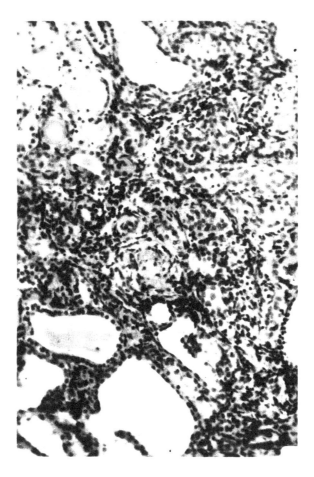

FIGURE 5B.    Section (approximately 400×) from a rat after
1000R showing a patch of more advanced arteriolar, glomerular, peritubular, and tubular fibrosis with less advancement of
this process on either side.

which the major calyces open. The ureters connect the renal pelvis with the urinary
bladder.

Each of these structures can be described as a unit, inasmuch as they have similar
basic structure. They are lined by stratified epithelium of a transitional type; that is,
its appearance and thickness vary with the degree of organ distention or contraction.
Since there is no basement membrane beneath the transitional epithelium, the underlying capillaries often penetrate or indent the deeper surface of the epithelium. The
lamina propria is composed largely of thin collagenous fibers and does not form pa-
pillae that indent the epithelium, as in the case of highly stratfied epithelium such as
epidermis. The lamina propria contains diffuse and occasionally nodular lymphoid
tissue. Beneath the lamina propria is a loose, more elastic connective tissue (submucosa) surrounded by layers of smooth muscle, which in turn are surrounded by adventitial connective tissue containing blood vessels, lymphatic vessels, and nerves.

Like other stratified epithelia, the stratified epithelium of the urinary bladder and
ureters contains a deep layer of proliferating vegetative intermitotic cells which supplies
cells for differentiation to replace the more differentiated superficial cells which are
being lost continuously. The vegetative intermitotic germinal cells are relatively sensi-

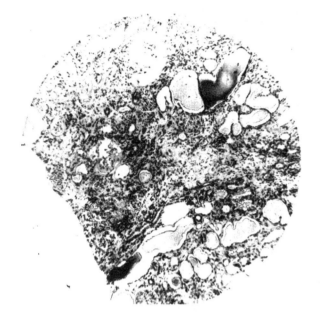

FIGURE 5D.   Section (approximately 100x) from a rat one year after irradiation, showing severe nephrosclerosis. (H. and E. stains.) (A and B from Wachholz, B. and Casarett, G. W., unpublished; C from Maier, J. G. and Casarett, G. W., U.S. Atomic Energy Commission Report UR-626, Washington, D.C., 1963; D from Casarett, G. W., *Radiat. Res. Suppl.*, 5, 246, 1964. With permission.)

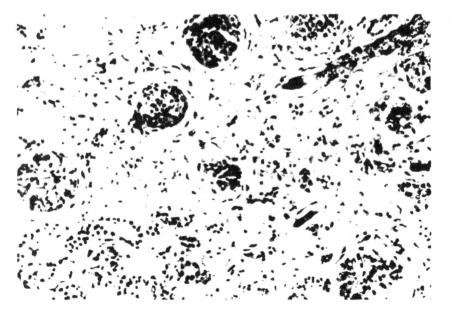

FIGURE 5C.   Section (approximately 400x) from a dog six months after 1000R, showing marked replacement fibrosis, with relative spatial concentration of glomeruli in various stages of degeneration and fibrosis.

tive to the direct destructive actions of ionizing radiation, as are the analogous cells of the epidermis.

In regard to the urinary bladder, in general, all that has been described about radiation effects on the skin and on mucosae with stratified (epidermoid) epithelium, with the exception of the special adnexal structures, applies essentially to radiation effects on the mucosa of the urinary bladder.

The ureteral epithelium, which is transitional stratified epithelium like that in the urinary bladder, is somewhat less sensitive to radiation than the bladder epithelium, possibly because of a lesser blood supply and oxygenation. With sufficient doses of radiation, however, radiation inflammation of the ureteral walls may be caused. Sequences of pathologic changes similar to those described for the skin also occur in the ureters.

Occlusion of the ureters may result from radiation damage to the ureteral walls, or extensive scar formation in the bladder may occlude the ureteral openings. In addition, ascending infection often results in ureteral and renal complications after irradiation. Ascending infection is often a result of ureteral obstruction.

Intensive irradiation of the pelvic region may cause relatively massive fibrosis throughout the pelvis, affecting the ureters and bladder, as well as other organs in the pelvic region.

Chapter 3

# CARDIOVASCULAR SYSTEM AND MUSCLE

The fine vasculature of the body, which is intimately incorporated into tissues and organs, has been considered generally in an earlier chapter on general radiation histopathology, and more specifically in the various chapters dealing with specific organs. The purpose in the present chapter is to consider the heart and the major blood vessels as organs, many of which contain fine vasculature (vasa vasorum), and also to consider muscle at the same time.

## I. HEART

The myocardium, the middle and major mass of the heart and the contractile layer of the heart wall, is a muscle composed of networks of striated muscle fibers which differ in some details from the structure of skeletal striated muscles (Figure 1A). Free endings of cardiac muscle fibers are generally absent, except in fibers in papillary muscles and in regions of atrial-ventricular apertures. Although the myofibrils are similar to those in the striated muscle fibers of skeletal muscle, the cytoplasm is relatively abundant, the mitochondria are much more numerous, and the nuclei are scattered irregularly in the interior, usually the axial part of the fiber, as contrasted with skeletal muscle fibers. The cardiac muscle fibers also contain short lines called intercalated discs running transverse to the long axis and usually bounded on both sides by Z discs. It is believed that the myofibrils stop at the intercalated discs. There is loose connective tissue in the narrow spaces of cardiac muscle, and the muscle fibers are surrounded by dense networks of blood capillaries. Lymphatic vessels are also abundant. The myocardium is analogous to the medial layer of blood vessels.

The regenerative ability of mature cardiac muscle cells is insignificant, if it exists at all. Injuries or pathologic damage to the cardiac muscle are repaired by secondary intention, that is by replacement fibrosis. Cardiac muscle cells are therefore classed as fixed postmitotic cells and are highly resistant to the direct destructive actions of radiation. The fine blood vessels, connective tissue cells, and mesothelium of the heart are only moderately resistant to radiation damage.

The endocardium, the thin layer of the heart wall, is analogous to the inner or intimal layer of blood vessels. It is lined at the lumenal surface by simple flat epithelium (ordinary vascular endothelium) continuous with the endothelium of the blood vessels entering and leaving the heart. The endothelium usually rests on a thin subendothelial layer of loose connective tissue, which in turn lies on a thick connective tissue layer containing numerous elastic elements and, in some places, in the peripheral parts of the layer, some smooth muscle fibers as well. Except for regions of papillary muscles and cordae tendinae, there is also a subendocardial layer of loose connective tissue between the endocardium and the myocardium. This subendocardial layer contains blood vessels, nerves, and branches of the heart's conduction system; the Purkinje fibers, a net of atypical muscle fibers of the impulse-conducting system, are found here, especially in the regions of interventricular septa.

The epicardium, the thin outer layer of the heart, is analogous to the outer or advential layer of the blood vessel walls and is composed of a single layer of mesothelial cells covering the free surface and resting on a thin layer of connective tissue containing networks of elastic fibers, many nervous elements, and blood vessels. The epicardium is essentially the visceral layer of the pericardium. The parietal layer of the pericardium

FIGURE 1B. Section (approximately 1000×; H. and E. stains) of rat cardiac muscle representing the picture of early radiation-induced interstitial edema.

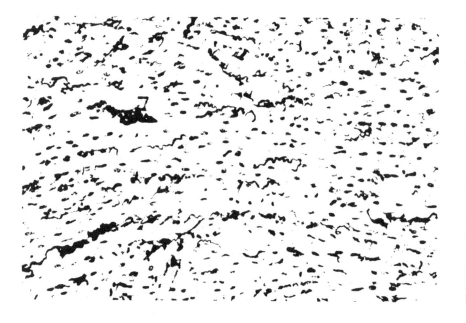

FIGURE 1. Sections of heart. A. Normal rat cardiac muscle (approximately 400×; silver, alcian blue, periodic acid Schiff stains).

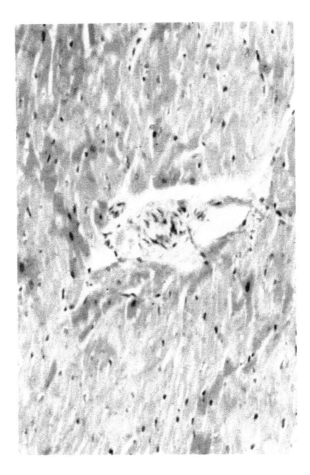

FIGURE 1C. Section (approximately 400×; H. and E. stains) of dog heart approximately 6 months after 1700R thoracic X-irradiation, showing sclerosis of a small artery and arteriole (center of picture) and subtle diffuse degenerative changes in cardiac muscle cells.

is a serous membrane, composed of a thin layer of connective tissue covered by a simple layer of mesothelial cells.

There has been relatively little radiohistopathologic study of the heart or large vessels in human subjects or animals of a definitive nature. Although there have been many reports in the literature concerning incidental observation of isolated responses of the cardiovascular system to radiation, there have been relatively few systematic studies.

Since the muscle cells of the heart are largely fixed postmitotic cells of long individual life span and correspondingly very resistant to the direct destructive actions of radiation, while the fine vasculature of the heart is only moderately radioresistant, the direct pathologic effects of irradiation of the heart involve primarily the fine vasculature, with secondary effects on connective tissue, and indirect effects on heart muscle.

Radiation-induced changes in the heart which have been reported include swelling of the fibers, loss of longitudinal and cross striations, homogenization of the sarcoplasm, delicate or coarse granulation of the sarcoplasm, and disappearance of protoplasm with persistence of hollow sarcolemma. Nuclei have been reported as showing pyknosis or hyperchromasia around the nuclear membrane, fragmentation, complete disintegration, or lysis. Small arterioles in the irradiated heart have shown thickened intima and degeneration and hyalinization of the media.

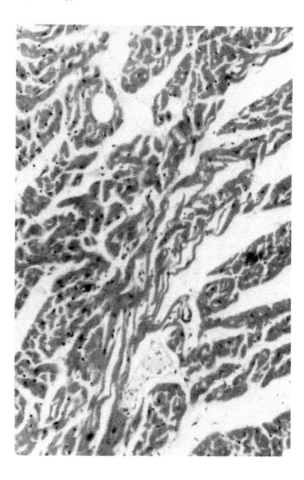

FIGURE 1D.   Section (approximately 400×; H. and E. stains) of dog heart approximately six months after 1700R thoracic X-irradiation, showing marked interstitial edema and diffuse degenerative changes in cardiac muscle cells associated with vascular changes in the vicinity. (A and B from Eddy, H. A. and Casarett, unpublished).

Early experimentalists reported that the heart muscle was relatively radioresistant histopathologically. Early structural changes in the myocardium were found only after high radiation doses, and were thought to be secondary to vascular damage. Warren's[202] summary of the histopathologic effects of radiation on the heart represents well the various observations of earlier workers and indicates that the obliterative vascular changes, together with aseptic necrosis and hyalin fibrosis, combine to form a fairly characteristic picture of cardiac damage resulting from irradiation of the heart. Pericardial changes have also been observed in radiotherapy patients, mostly in cases of irradiation of juxtapericardial neoplasms.

Gross and microscopic evidence has indicated that the right auricle and ventricle in man, the dog, and the rat are more severely damaged by ionizing radiation than are the left auricle and ventricle. Further study is required to elucidate the reasons for this difference.

As in other organs, early changes after large radiation doses include temporary edema, which in muscle separates fibers (Figure 1B).

The following description of the early histopathologic effects of single doses of radiation on the heart is based on the work of Leach and Sugiura[192] on rats given single doses of 1,500 to 20,000 rads to the heart region. The pericardium, myocardium, endocardium, and coronary vessels showed no microscopic abnormalities in rats killed at various times within 68 days after irradiation with doses of 5000 rads or less. With a dose of 7500 rads, rats sacrificed 7 to 80 days after irradiation showed no significant changes, except for mild thickening of the walls of coronary vessels and irregular staining of muscle fibers at 80 days. Sections of the hearts of rats killed 8 to 73 days after irradiation with 10,000 rads showed a normal pericardium, myocardium, and endocardium, except for very small areas of round cell infiltration in the myocardium. However, the hearts of rats that died spontaneously after this dose (at 23 and 26 days) showed intercellular edema of the myocardium, with the presence of fibrin, marked capillary engorgement, and some regions of capillary hemorrhage. There were also many areas of diffuse round cell infiltration. The muscle fibers were thinner than normal, and in some the cross striations were indistinct. Many of the muscle cell nuclei in one of these rats showed swelling, stained poorly, and were slightly to moderately pyknotic. After a dose of 20,000 rads, all five of the rats so exposed died within 6 to 14 days. In three of these rats there was mild subpericardial edema and congestion, with mild round cell infiltration. The pericardial endothelium was intact, and the endocardium was normal. In the myocardium of all five there was diffuse edema, capillary congestion, capillary hemorrhage, and moderate to severe round cell infiltration. The myocardial fibers were often shrunken, and the nuclei in many areas were slightly swollen or had become pyknotic, and in some cases were undergoing dissolution. The walls of the coronary vessels in many areas were thinned out and vacuolated.

As to later histopathologic changes, the radiation damage of fine vasculature of the heart may progress slowly to fibrosis of small coronary arteries (Figure 1C) and associated gradual degeneration of areas of heart muscle (Figure 1D). These processes may progress to more severe vascular and circulatory impairment, heart muscle degeneration and necrosis, and replacement fibrosis long after irradiation, the rate, degree, and extent depending on the dose and dose rate (Figure 2).

The spectrum of heart disease observed following irradiation is as follows:

1. Acute pericarditis. Increased vascular permeability, plasmatic transudation, fine vascular obstruction, and acute inflammation.
2. Chronic pericarditis. Pericardial effusion and fibrosis; constrictive pericarditis associated with myocardial fibrosis and endocardial fibroelastosis, with adhesions. Cardiac tamponade from constricting fibrosis; thick pericardium.
3. Coronary artery disease with myocardial infarction.
4. Mitral valve insufficiency and myocardial disease.

## II. SKELETAL MUSCLE

Striated skeletal muscle fibers are large, long, cylindrical, multinucleated cells with tapered ends. In striated muscle bundles, the muscle fibers, although closely parallel to each other and held together by connective tissue, are independent of one another. Several primary muscle bundles are combined to form secondary bundles, several secondary bundles are combined to form tertiary bundles, etc. The thick layer of connective tissue at the periphery of the muscles extends into the spaces between the bundles of muscle fibers and between the individual muscle fibers of primary muscle bundles. Blood vessels are abundant. Capillaries surround and form a dense network along the individual muscle fibers.

The striated muscle fiber is striated both longitudinally and transversely by thin

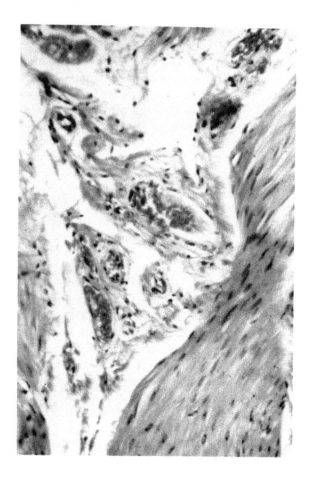

FIGURE 2.   Sections showing late effects of X-irradiation in
heart and skeletal muscle. A. Section of dog heart (approximately 400×) showing advanced sclerotic changes in fine vasculature.

cross-striated myofibrils. The muscle fiber is contained by a cell membrane (sarcolemma). The numerous nuclei of the muscle fiber are usually found in the layer of
sarcoplasm beneath the sarcolemma.

As a result of muscular activity, skeletal muscles increase in volume by enlargement
of the existing fibers through an increase in the sarcoplasm. Large areas of damage in
the skeletal muscle tissue are healed by replacement fibrosis, with the formation of
scars. Smaller defects may be healed by regenerative replacement of lost or defective
parts of muscle fibers from the remaining viable parts (nuclei and sarcoplasm) of these
fibers. The viable nuclei in the defective fiber, together with their surrounding sarcoplasm, become separate cells (sarcoblasts or myoblasts) within the sarcoplasm; the ends
of the fibers near the region go toward the damaged region as muscular buds; the
sarcoblasts enlarge, multiply, digest the degenerate fibers, fuse in groups and form
new fiber within the reticulum of the old fiber.

Although this form of regeneration includes nuclear (sarcoblast) multiplication, the
regeneration involves repair or growth of preexisting fibers rather than multiplication
of the whole muscle cell (fiber). Therefore the muscle cell or fiber as a whole behaves
as a fixed postmitotic cell, although its nuclei may behave in a reverting postmitotic
manner when the fiber is damaged. In any case, mature striated muscle cells are relatively resistant to the direct cytocidal actions of radiation.

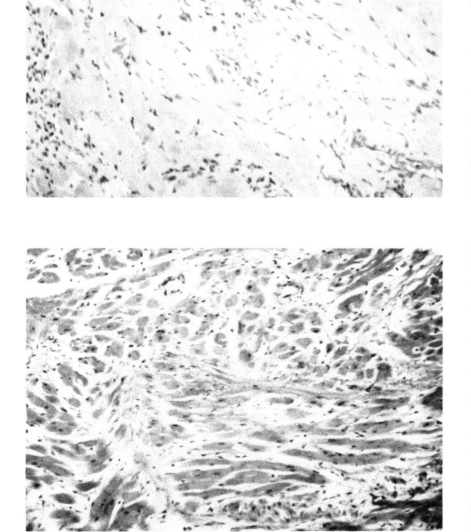

FIGURE 2C. Fibrosis in rat myocardium (approximately 400×). (H. and E. stains).

FIGURE 2B. Section of dog heart (approximately 400×) showing an area of degeneration and active fibrosis in the myocardium, with sclerotic thickening of fine vasculature.

There has been little systematic study of the histopathologic sequence of events in muscles as organs after various doses of radiation. Degeneration and necrosis and fibrous replacement of muscle within or near other organs that have undergone severe nonselective radionecrosis secondary to vascular occlusion have been mentioned in preceding chapters and in many pieces of literature as incidental findings.

Because of the relatively great resistance of mature muscle cells to the direct cytocidal actions of radiation, massive radiation doses (50,000 rads) are required to cause early necrosis of muscles, and this inevitably involves early severe disruption of the fine vasculature and microcirculation, with increased capillary permeability, edema, and inflammation, through which much of the early organ damage is mediated. After such massive doses, the interstitial edema and inflammation may begin within an hour or so and rapidly increase, with the occurrence of small hemorrhages. Muscle fibers become swollen and hyalin in appearance, with loss of striations, and within a day or two after irradiation many muscle fibers may rupture. Necrosis and thrombosis of arteries may develop rapidly, and gross muscle necrosis may become apparent within a few days. Macrophages become numerous in the necrotic muscle, in addition to the granulocytes of the acute inflammatory exudate.

With decreasing doses, such early changes in muscle occur to a lesser degree until, at large but not massive doses, the acute edematous and inflammatory expressions of vascular damage and the early changes in muscle fibers secondary to these events are more moderate and transient. However, even with doses which do not cause these early changes in muscle fibers, but which do cause substantial degrees of acute interstitial edema and inflammation, the associated vascular damage and connective tissue reactions may progress in time to cause delayed secondary degeneration, atrophy or necrosis, and fibrosis of irradiated muscles (Figure 3). The larger the dose, within an effective dose range, the earlier this delayed effect on muscles tends to occur, depending upon the rate of progression of the vascular obliterative changes and circulatory impairment.

## III. SMOOTH MUSCLE

Smooth muscle is closely related to ordinary connective tissue and is located chiefly in the internal organs, as described in previous chapters. Smooth muscle cells (fibers) are usually long and spindle-shaped, and sometimes branched. The nucleus is located in the middle or widest part of the cell. The cytoplasm contains fine myofibrils (filaments) running parallel and lengthwise through the cell, and the sarcoplasm is found between the fibrils. In smooth muscle bundles the cells are arranged with the thick middle part of the cell adjacent to the thin ends of neighboring cells, and the connective tissue fibers around muscle cells bind the muscle cells together. Between muscle bundles or layers there is loose collagenous and elastic connective tissue which contains a vascular network.

Mitosis has been reported in smooth muscle cells in the vicinity of organ damage. However, the infrequency and small degree of such reported findings, the fact that necrosis of smooth muscle is often observed to heal largely by scar formation, plus the possibility that the formation of new smooth muscle cells arising from perivascular mesenchymal cells could be mistaken for division of muscle cells, suggest that most, if not all, formed smooth muscle cells behave as fixed postmitotic cells. However, the possibility is left that some smooth muscle cells may behave as reverting postmitotic cells under special conditions. In any case, mature smooth muscle cells are relatively resistant to the direct cytocidal actions of radiation.

As is pointed out in the other chapters dealing with specific organ systems, smooth

FIGURE 3. Section of human skeletal muscle under skin about a year after irradiation incidental to radiotherapy, showing fibrosis, chronic inflammation, and sclerosis of fine vasculature. (H. and E. stains; magnification approximately 200×.)

muscle undergoes degeneration in the wake of vascular damage, edema, and inflammation.

## IV. BLOOD VESSELS

Although the diameter of the lumen of an artery decreases as it proceeds distally from the heart, the sum of the lumenal diameters of its branches gradually increases. The endothelial lining is continuous from the heart to the capillaries, but the other layers of the vessel walls, particularly the medial layer, are different in composition as they go from the heart to arterioles, according to the size and functional variables of the vessels. With respect to the composition of the medial layer, the smallest arteries (arterioles) are predominantly muscular, as are the small-to-medium-sized arteries, whereas the large arteries, for example the aorta, are predominantly elastic. However, there are no sharp limits to such arbitrary divisions for the medium-sized arteries. Furthermore, the change from muscular to elastic types or vice versa, although sometimes rather abrupt, as in the lower aorta and its branches, is usually gradual, with mixed types being intermediate between the two extremes, for example, external carotid, axillary, and common iliac arteries.

In arterioles (about 0.04 to 0.3 mm in diameter) the wall is thicker, relative to the lumenal diameter, than in any other blood vessel. The intimal layer is thin and contains little or no obvious subendothelial tissue. The underlying internal elastic membrane is sometimes vague. The media is the thickest layer and is purely muscular, consisting of one to several layers of smooth muscle cells. The adventitial layer is thinner than the media; it is composed of fibroelastic tissue, and it lacks a definite external elastic membrane.

Small and medium-sized arteries as a group include the muscular types, most of the arteries which have been given names, and all those which have not been given names. These arteries contain a subendothelial connective tissue layer, however thin, and a prominent internal elastic membrane. The medial layer is thick, and the larger medium-sized vessels may contain some elastic tissue or, in the largest of these vessels, even some elastic membranes, as well as small amounts of collagenous connective tissue. The adventitia may be thick, although thinner than the media, and contains an elastic layer or external elastic membrane adjacent to the media, surrounded externally by collagenous connective tissue.

The group of large arteries includes all arteries of the elastic type, for example, the aorta and its largest main branches. In these vessels, the lumen is relatively large in comparison with the wall thickness, the endothelial cells are not as elongated or flattened as in small vessels, the subendothelial connective tissue layer is relatively thick and contains many elastic fibers, the thick media is composed chiefly of elastic and collagenous connective tissue, and the adventitia is relatively thin.

The elastic arteries are conducting arteries in which the elastic tissue expands to absorb some of the pulse beat of the heart and temporarily store some of the energy involved. In the return of the stretched walls during refilling of the heart, the elastic tissue releases kinetic energy and maintains a more constant pressure and a smoother, less interruptive flow of blood. The muscular arteries are distributing arteries which, under the nervous control of their muscular medial layers, can regulate the quantities of blood brought to various organs and tissues according to need by contracting or dilating. The arterioles, with their relatively thick muscular walls and narrow lumen, play a prime role in controlling the local flow of blood in tissues and in controlling systemic blood pressure, being responsible for most of the fall in blood pressure within tissues and organs.

Owing perhaps to the wear and tear of constant mechanical activity, the arterial system, including the heart, seems to deteriorate by usage more than any other organ systems. The process of differentiation passes into progressive aging changes of a regressive nature which lead to arteriosclerosis. The elastic arteries, especially the aorta, show the effect of use chiefly in irregular thickening of the intima, with subsequent degenerative changes in the media, and show much greater change with age than do the muscular arteries. In medium-sized arteries of the muscular type, the main changes are calcification in the media and intimal thickening and fibrosis. Eventually the small arteries and arterioles show important changes in structure and number with age.

The lumenal diameter of an artery is less than that of the corresponding vein or groups of veins, and the vein wall is thinner, less rigid, more easily collapsible and less elastic than that of the artery. Muscular and elastic tissues are less well developed, and connective tissue is more prominent in veins as compared with arteries. The division of veins into small (venules), medium, and large caliber veins with respect to generalized structural details is less clear than with arteries, because size and structure are not well correlated, and there is greater individual variability. Also, the intimal, medial, and adventitial boundaries are often not distinct.

The venules, which are about 0.2 to 1.0 mm in diameter, have an intimal layer composed only of endothelium, without subendothelial connective tissue or an internal elastic membrane, a thin medial layer consisting of one to a few layers of muscle cells, and a relatively thick adventitial layer of homogenous connective tissue. In the small and medium-sized veins (1 to 10 mm in diameter) there is sometimes a thin layer of subendothelial connective tissue and sometimes a network of elastic fibers in the intima, the bundles of smooth muscles are separated by collagenous fibers and elastic networks in the media, and there is a relatively thick fibroelastic adventitial layer sometimes containing smooth muscle. In the large veins, e.g., the vena cava, portal vein, and main tributaries, the subendothelial connective tissue is thicker and may contain some bundles of smooth muscle, there is sometimes a thin internal elastic membrane, and the thick adventitial connective tissue layer usually contains bundles of smooth muscle. The valves which appear in many of the small or medium-sized veins are formed by foldings of the intimal layer.

The walls of all arteries and veins having a caliber larger than 1 mm contain their own blood vessels (vasa vasorum). In the arteries they do not go farther than the external regions of the medial layer, but in the veins they are usually more abundant and in some cases run as deep into the wall as the intimal layer. The venous vessels of the vasa vasorum often empty into the lumens of the blood vessels which they serve. The larger arteries and veins also contain lymphatic vessels which drain into perivascular vessels.

Injuries to blood or lymph capillaries may be repaired by primary intention, that is by regeneration of endothelial cells. New growth of these capillaries when required, e.g., in wound healing or neoplasia, begins with budding or outgrowth of endothelial sprouts into regenerating or neoplastic areas. Solid outgrowths become hollow. With fibroblasts at hand and with differentiation of myoblasts, additional vascular wall layers may then be developed around the endothelial tubes to form larger vessels as required. These processes are generally slower in lymphatic vessels and sometimes do not occur. Severe damage to the endothelium of large vessels or damage to other layers of the walls as well, may become repaired by secondary intention to some extent, that is by replacement fibrosis.

The endothelial cells of vessels behave as reverting postmitotic cells, but presumably because of the wear and tear of blood flow, blood pressure, contraction, and dilatation, may undergo relatively more frequent divisions than many other types of postmitotic cells. They are moderately sensitive to the direct destructive action of radiation, as are active fibroblasts. Smooth muscle cells are largely long-lived postmitotic cells and are highly resistant to the direct destructive actions of radiation.

Experimental work on dogs[193] given X-irradiation to localized segments of the abdominal aorta and examined histologically at intervals from 2 to 48 weeks has shown that the irradiation results in aortic arteriosclerosis in the irradiated sites which is qualitatively indistinguishable from the aortic arteriosclerosis occurring eventually in a natural fashion in dogs. Large doses caused less extreme lesions than did smaller doses, an indication that the larger doses, though presumably causing greater degrees of initial damage, inhibited the full development of the lesions within the period of observation. The degree of arteriosclerosis increased with time after irradiation. The cause of this arteriosclerosis, according to these authors, may be a selective injury of the internal elastic membrane, leading to intimal fibrosis and plaque formation. In this study, the earliest observed radiation lesion was located in the internal fenestrated membrane, and the authors stressed the intimate genetic relationship of this membrane to the enveloping mucopolysaccharide matrix.

Physiologic studies of the irradiated nonliving aortic intima have indicated the functional importance and the radiation sensitivity of the subendothelial gel filtration layer or basement membrane covering the fenestrated elastic membrane on the lumenal side.[190] First, direct evidence of radiation effects has been found in the instantaneous drop of the injection pressure in the aortic wall during irradiation; this pressure drop demonstrates an increased permeability to water caused by depolymerization of the mucopolysaccharides in the matrix and possibly in membranous structures in close relation to the matrix. The possibility exists that radiochemical changes in the matrix substance may cause changes in the development of its fibrous and laminar structures, e.g., in the basement membrane. Impairment of the function of the aortic basement membrane or gel filtration layer by irradiation was also shown by the deeper and faster rate of diffusion of dyes through the endothelium and into the wall of irradiated pieces

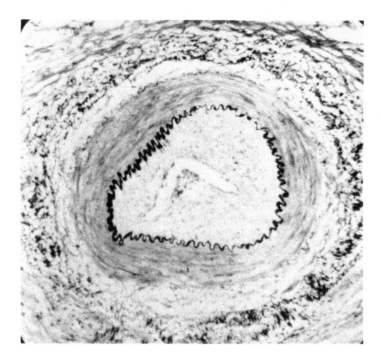

FIGURE 4.    Section of human mesenteric artery about 6 months after irradiation incidental to radiotherapy, showing marked subendothelial (intimal) connective tissue proliferation, marked narrowing of the lumen, and medial and adventitial fibrosis. (H. and E. stains; magnification approximately 200×.) (From Rubin, P. and Casarett, G. W., *Clinical Radiation Pathology*, W. B. Saunders, Philadelphia, 1968. With permission.)

of excised aorta (cow, pig, sheep) after a dose of 2000 rads. Similar results were observed 30 min after intravenous injection of a dye in rats just after whole-body irradiation with doses of 1000 to 3000 rads.

Studies of the effects of $^{60}$Co gamma rays on isolated surviving arteries (swine and dog carotid arteries in vivo) and their vasa vasorum, by means of an angioplethismal method,[198] have shown marked early reductions in blood flow in the vasa vasorum in the carotids of swine (70% decrease) and dogs (50% decrease) exposed to 9390 rads in 15 min. Less marked, but significant reductions in blood flow were observed after lower doses of 3000, 2085, and 1500 rads.

Medium-sized muscular arteries also show degenerative intimal, medial, and adventitial changes after irradiation, although these and the large arteries are not as severely damaged as are arterioles and capillaries. The large and medium-sized veins show similar change, but perhaps not to the degree that arteries are affected. Similar, but lesser effects may also be observed in lymphatic vessels of comparable sizes.

The repair of acute injury to the blood vessel walls by secondary intention (fibrosis) leaves a residuum of advanced degrees of vascular sclerosis, as compared with nonirradiated vessels in individuals of similar age. In addition to the narrowing and obliteration of the vasa vasorum, there may be excessive proliferation of medial elements in the larger vessels and excessive proliferation of subendothelial connective tissue and/or endothelium, with narrowing of the lumens (Figure 4). Such changes may be slowly progressive with time, of the nature of endarteritis obliterans in some vessels, and tending in the direction of obliteration of the lumens in some areas.

Even in the absence of marked radiation effects on the larger blood vessels in the acute and subacute periods, the more subtle damage and progressive sclerosis of the vasa vasorum or other elements of the walls of large vessels may lead after many years to significant lesions of the large vessels. The chronic residual progressive deterioration of irradiated vessels reduces their resilience and their resistance to further irradiation, damage, infection, or stress. For example, it has been shown[179] that irradiation of blood vessels sensitizes them to damage from subsequent developing hypertension, in comparison with previously nonirradiated vessels.

The effects of radiation on the fine vasculature have already been discussed generally in an earlier chapter concerned with radiation histopathology, and more specifically in the various chapters dealing with specific organs. It was pointed out that the damage to the peripheral parts of the vascular system is diffuse, though irregular in degree, and is probably caused by a combination of the direct effects of radiation on the component cells of the blood vessels (especially the endothelial cells), indirect effects associated with damage of associated tissues, and the consequent inflammatory process. The relative importance of each of these changes in contributing to the damage and dysfunction in the fine vasculature following irradiation remains to be determined. The special importance of the fine vasculature in radiation effects was pointed out, in relation to its intimate relationship with the respiration and metabolism of dependent parenchymal cells and the relatively easy occludability of lumens of this vasculature by wall thickening, as compared with the larger vessels which serve only as gross plumbing and gross mechanical regulators of hemodynamics.

Nevertheless, the large blood vessels, having their own system of fine vasculature, may suffer radiation damage secondary to effects on these systems, much as do other types of organs. Ionizing radiation may interfere with the nutrition of the walls of large blood vessels by damaging the fine blood vessels serving their walls. Damage to the vasa vasorum may be irregular, although widespread, as is the case in fine vasculature of other organs, and this may be the reason for the segmental or irregular radiation damage observed in large blood vessels. The precise mechanism of radiation damage to large vessels is not yet completely clear.

Chapter 4

# MAJOR DIGESTIVE AND ENDOCRINE GLANDS

The major digestive glands (salivary glands, liver, and pancreas) and endocrine glands (pancreas, thyroid, parathyroid, adrenal, pituitary) to be discussed in this chapter (gonads to be discussed in the next chapter) contain parenchymal tissues composed of reverting postmitotic radioresistant cells.

## I. MAJOR DIGESTIVE GLANDS

### A. Salivary Glands

The large salivary glands (parotid, submaxillary or submandibular, and sublingual glands) have excretory ducts opening into the oral cavity. These are compound branching tubuloalveolar merocrine glands, serous or mucous or mixed (Figure 1). The gland cells and duct cells behave essentially as reverting postmitotic cells in that under normal conditions only occasional mitotic figures are observed, and they are relatively resistant to the direct destructive actions of radiation. However, they are capable of dividing to replace lost cells, provided they are supported by an adequate circulation. Regeneration is accomplished by proliferation of secretory and duct cells. Blood vessels follow the ducts and form abundant capillary networks around the secretory structures and terminal ducts.

The parotid gland is purely serous, i.e., its secretion is watery and albuminous. The parotid secretion is especially important in the contribution of digestive enzymes to the saliva, including ptyalin or amylase, which converts starch to maltose, and maltase, which converts maltose to glucose. The secretory end structures (alveoli or acinae) are at the ends or sides of the secretory tubules and are lined by cuboidal serous cells, usually a single layer. There are secretory capillaries between alveolar cells extending from the alveolar lumen to the basement membrane.

The intralobular secretory ducts are lined with simple reverting postmitotic radioresistant cells. The relatively large interlobular excretory ducts are lined at first by simple columnar radioresistant epithelium, then by pseudostratified radioresistant epithelium in some of the main trunks, and by stratified epithelium near the main outlet to the oral cavity. This stratified epithelium, like that of the oral mucosa with which it merges, contains vegetative intermitotic cells in the basal layer which are relatively radiosensitive.

The submaxillary gland is a mixed (serous-mucous) gland containing many more serous alveoli than mixed alveoli. Mucous cell cytoplasm elaborates the protein mucigen which when secreted and mixed with water becomes mucin or, with other additions, mucus. Secretory capillaries, such as occur between serous cells, are lacking in mucous alveoli.

The sublingual salivary gland, a composite of glands, is a mixed gland more variable in composition than the other salivary glands. The secretory end pieces of a sublingual gland are branching tubules in which the mucous cells are much more numerous than serous cells. The secretory tubules are purely mucous or mixed, and even the serous cells have semimucoid characteristics.

Contrary to expectations on the basis of the classification of the parenchymal cells of the salivary glands as reverting postmitotic cells, the salivary glands appear to be moderately radiosensitive functionally, and in parts (especially serous portions) histopathologically. Presently available data on the sequence of events in these glands im-

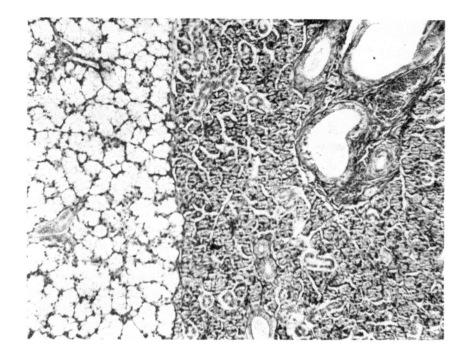

FIGURE 1.    Section of normal rat submandibular salivary gland showing a serous portion on the left and a mucous portion on the right. (H. and E. stains; magnification approximately 200×.)

mediately after irradiation, with respect to all their components, are insufficient to provide a definitive explanation of the precise mechanisms of the radiation effects. These data and their interpretation vary among different investigators, and the variations are partly related to differences in species, conditions of investigation and the controls, criteria of effect, consideration of various organ components, radiation factors, and postirradiation observation times.

There has been relatively little attention directed specifically toward an adequate evaluation of the sequential effects of radiation of the fine vasculature of the salivary glands, despite the known moderate radiosensitivity of the endothelium of the fine vasculature and the increased permeability, interstitial edema, and perivascular inflammation that occurs shortly after moderate doses of radiation. However, the bulk of presently available information obtained from the experimental animals and human specimens suggests that the changes observed in the parenchymal epithelium after irradiation are largely secondary to changes in the fine vasculature, edema, and inflammation. Also, there may be an involvement of autoimuune reactions which may help to explain why the glands are moderately radioresponsive.

The rapid and marked swelling of the salivary glands that begins within a day after irradiation may be attributable at least partly to changes in the endothelium of the fine vasculature, congestion and increased permeability of capillaries, interstitial edema, acute inflammatory cell infiltration, and sometimes partly to narrowing of excretory ducts by the pressure of edema and inflammation, swelling of duct lining, or plugging of lumens by mucus. Such changes may be expected to inhibit or otherwise alter the function of secretory cells, to cause collapse or disconnection of some of them from their bases, and, if severe, to cause degeneration and necrosis of cells.

Kashima et al.[210] have provided valuable histopathologic observations of specimens of the various human salivary glands obtained surgically 24 hr after irradiation with large single doses (1000 to 2000 rads). In general, there was a close parallel between the location and degree of the acute inflammatory cell infiltration and the degenerative changes in the glandular epithelium. Both of these changes were limited largely to serous portions of the glands. The changes were regarded as dose-dependent. The acute inflammatory changes consisted of infiltration by polymorphonuclear leukocytes, eosinophilic leukocytes, and a few plasma cells along interlobular septa (where in some glands there was frank zonal suppuration) and around acini; sometimes these cells were seen among the granules of degenerating serous cells. There was also purulent exudate in the lumens of intercalated, interlobular and excretory ducts which appeared to be composed of degenerating polymorphonuclear leukocytes and degenerating acinous cells. The degenerative changes in the acini and cells of serous glands included a vagueness of acinar outlines, basilar vacuoles or spaces seeming to rupture cells and cleave them from the basement membrane, pyknosis of some cells, pooling of zymogen granules of the acini, and in some glands a reduction in the number of zymogen granules.

In the same study it was reported that elevation of body temperature was infrequent, leukocytosis rare, and evidence of activation of a bacterial or viral agent absent in the histologic studies and the clinical course. The authors offered these observations as support for the conclusion that the irradiation of the salivary glands was causally related to the hyperamylasemia they observed. They pointed out that the mechanism of the tissue reaction is unexplained, but suggested that the observation that the serous cells exhibited greatest damage indicates that it is in these cells that the primary damage occurs. They attributed the appearance of the salivary amylase in the serum to the disruption of serous cells or changes in cell permeability with release of intracellular amylase into the circulation, and they regarded the marked inflammatory cell infiltration into the gland as a response to serous cell degeneration.

A difference of opinion on one aspect of this explanation should be noted here. The primary effect of irradiation in this mechanism need not be a direct effect on the serous cells. The primary effect may be on the endothelium of the fine vasculature, with resulting increased capillary permeability and interstitial edema. It is not known whether serous cells are more susceptible than mucous cells to degeneration caused by such changes in the fine vasculature or by interstitial edema. However, the fact that serous acini have secretory capillaries between acinous cells, extending from the acinar lumen to the basement membrane, whereas mucous glands do not, raises the possibility that the serous gland secretion, including amylase, could enter altered capillaries even without prior destruction or damage of serous cells. If this caused the observed inflammatory cell infiltration into the serous gland regions, the degeneration of serous gland epithelium could then have been secondary to the inflammation. If this proved to be the case, the lack of observed mucous cell degeneration could be explained on the basis that the mucous gland secretion did not enter the altered capillaries. The inflammatory cell infiltration described by Kashima et al. is compatible with an autoimmune antigen-antibody reaction.

Following the early changes in salivary glands after moderate to large radiation doses, the inflammatory cell infiltration becomes characterized by a predominence of lymphoid cells and plasma cells over polymorphonuclear cells, and the process of interstitial fibrosis begins with the appearance of increased numbers of active fibroblasts. After moderate doses, the structural alterations in the glandular epithelium may be relatively minor and subtle, especially in the mucous components, may vary in different fields, and may include changes in size, shape, and staining characteristics of some cells, collapse of some cells, indistinct cell outlines, vacuolization of cytoplasm, separation of some cells from the basement membrane by edema, reduction in the number of zymogen granules in some cells, pooling of zymogen granules in some acini, and

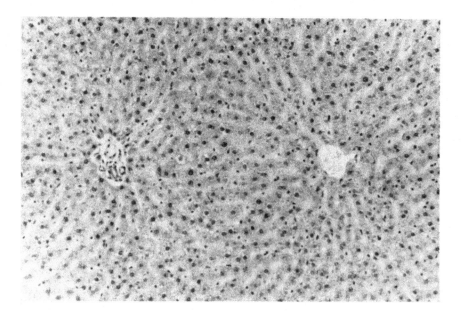

FIGURE 2.    Section of normal rat liver showing a centrolobular vein at the right and a portal area (branches of portal vein, hepatic artery, and bile duct) at the periphery of the lobule(s) at the left. (H. and E. stains; magnification approximately 200×.)

degeneration of some nuclei (pyknosis, karyorrhexis, chromatolysis). These earlier changes are more prominent in serous gland epithelium than in mucous gland epithelium, and the epithelium of the ducts is least affected, especially that of the excretory ducts.

As time progresses after relatively large doses there may be progressive degeneration and loss of acinous epithelium and acini (with progressive glandular atrophy) concomitant with progressive degeneration of fine vasculature and increase in interstitial fibrosis. These progressive changes are more advanced at comparable times in serous acini than in mucous acini, but mucous acini are eventually affected progressively.

Depending on the degree of initial damage, there may be more or less evidence of regeneration of acinous cells, which tends to be transient or abortive at high dose levels. However, these attempts are followed by the continued progression of the degenerative processes. Recovery of the ducts from initial damage, which is less than that suffered by the acini, is usually more successful, and later changes in these ductal structures, as well as in acini, seem to be secondary to the progressive changes in the fine vasculature and interstitial connective tissue. At times, the ductal epithelium may become hyperplastic or show squamous metaplasia. With progressive loss of acini, the intercalated ducts may produce some functional acini, and the ducts and the secretory tubules become relatively increased in proportion in the remaining glandular mass.

## B. Liver

The liver is essentially a compound tubular, serous, merocrine gland which is highly modified by replacement of tubules by branching and anastomosing cords or plates of epithelial cells and reorganization of the parenchyma into lobular units (Figure 2).

The liver parenchyma is divided into many small lobules. An hepatic lobule consists of plates or cords of liver cells, usually in a single layer, separated by blood sinusoids (lined by endothelial cells and phagocytic Kuppfer cells) arranged in radial fashion from the axis of the lobule (the central vein) to the perilobular capsular connective tissue which contains the portal system or portal canals (branches of the hepatic artery, portal vein, bile duct, and lymphatic vessels). The sinusoids join the perilobular blood vessels with the central vein. The central veins join to form larger veins, which in turn join to form branches of the hepatic veins. Between the cells of the hepatic plates are bile capillaries, which drain toward the periphery of the lobule into a bile duct in the portal region. The bile ducts are lined by simple cuboidal or low columnar epithelium.

The periphery of the lobule is the most active part of the lobule functionally. The middle or paracentral zone is less active, and the central zone (zone of repose) is functional upon extraordinary demand. The liver performs many functions despite the morphologic similarity of all hepatic cells. The secretory product of the exocrine gland aspect of the liver is bile, including bile acids, bile pigments, cholesterol, lecithin, fats, urea, etc.. The liver excretes bile pigment derived from hemoglobin through the action of the reticuloendothelial system, excretes urea formed in the liver from the breakdown of amino acids as a byproduct of protein metabolism, and excretes cholesterol, lecithin, and fats into the bile. The liver stores blood, stores glycogen and releases it to the blood as glucose (the so-called endocrine function), stores vitamins (especially vitamins A and B), enzymes, hormones, and fat, and can transform fats into carbohydrates. The liver is one of the organs which stores heparin. It also synthesizes protein, such as fibrinogen, which is secreted to the blood, and it forms an antianemic substance which stimulates the regeneration of red blood cells. The phagocytic Kuppfer cells, like macrophages of the reticuloendothelial system, remove particulate matter, such as bacteria, defunct blood elements, and foreign particles from the blood stream, and help to establish immunities.

The liver has two afferent blood supplies, one mostly venous (75%) from the portal veins and the other arterial (25%) from the hepatic areteries. Each hepatic cell is exposed to blood on two surfaces.

Hepatic cells and the cells of the simple epithelial lining of the intrahepatic and extrahepatic bile ducts and the gall bladder behave as reverting postmitotic cells and are relatively resistant to the direct destructive actions of radiation. They do not divide regularly, and hence mitotic figures are rare at any given time under normal conditions. However, they may respond to excessive loss of cells by dividing to replace them. Degenerating or dying cells are somewhat more common than dividing cells in the normal liver, and probably some of the cell loss is compensated by an increase in size of some of the remaining cells. When an extensive loss of liver tissue occurs, as from toxic agents or surgery, the remaining liver tissue shows a marked capacity for regenerating promptly to replace the lost tissue. Hepatic cells proliferate and enlarge, and new lobules bud from older lobules. There is also proliferation of bile ducts, and some new hepatic cells may differentiate from proliferating bile duct epithelium.

It is possible also that the great vascularity of the liver, with 75% of the blood supply being venous, and with its blood circulation through sinusoidal vessels of relatively large caliber and lined by radioresistant phagocytic cells rather than through narrow capillaries lined by endothelial cells alone, may confer some added degree of radioresistance in terms of radiation effects that are commonly secondary to vascular effects in other types of organs.

The bulk of the histopathologic evidence obtained from liver specimens from human beings and experimental animals after irradiation, although sparse and far from definitive, supports the view that necrosis and atrophy of hepatic cells caused by irradiation is largely secondary to radiation damage to the small blood vessels in the liver.

Early (acute) histopathologic changes after large radiation doses (greater than 2000 rads) include severe sinusoidal congestion, hyperemia or hemorrhage, some atrophy of the central hepatic cells, mild dilatation of the central veins with erythrocytes, and scattered fat vacuoles in hepatic cells in the hyperemic regions. Subsequent early vascular changes include damage and loss of endothelial cells, thickening of subintimal connective tissue, and formation of loose cellular and fibrillar tissue (fibroblasts and collagen fibers) which sometimes fills lumens of centrolobular veins. These centrolobular vein changes may be followed by degeneration and atrophy of centrolobular hepatic cords.

With passing time, in man the changes in the centrolobular veins (and also portal area arterioles) progress in degree and extent (number of veins involved), with increasing compactness and contraction of collagen fibers. Obliterative changes may become advanced in many small efferent veins. With time there may be also some increase in collagen fibers surrounding the veins (perivascular fibrosis) in the altered lobular centers and extending among the hepatic cell cords (interstitial fibrosis). Venous lumens tend to become completely obliterated and lobular organization less distinct.

Reed and Cox[222] likened the appearance of the altered hepatic lobules to that of hepatic veno-occlusive disease in man arising under other conditions. They concluded that the vascular lesion was an early result of irradiation and that the hyperemia and hepatic cell loss or atrophy were secondary to the vascular obstruction in the small branches of the hepatic veins. Dose size permitting, there may be sufficient recovery of an effective circulatory system in the damaged regions to lead to considerable restoration of hepatic cells and hepatic architecture, probably by means of the development of collateral circulatory channels. In addition to the progressive fibrous obliteration of the small branches of the hepatic veins, there may also be some thickening of the small portal vein branches and focal intimal thickening of the small arteries.

There is insufficient definitive information on the earliest, intermediate, and late effects of radiation on the liver to provide a clear picture of the complete pathogenetic sequence of events.

Ariel[214] performed detailed experiments to investigate the early (few days to 20 days) effects of single doses (300 to 100,000 rads) of X-rays after partial irradiation of the livers of rabbits. After 300 rads, the essential findings within a week were mild intercellular hepatic edema and mild engorgement in the smaller blood vessels, with slight separation of the liver cords, most marked at three days, and in the central parts of the lobule and near larger blood vessels; these changes almost completely disappeared by the seventh day.

After 3000 rads, with study for a week, the findings included at 12 hours marked polymorphonuclear leukocytes mostly in the portal spaces and to a lesser extent elsewhere, dilatation and congestion of many blood vessels, slight edema, rare portal hemorrhage, and increase in the number and size of fibroblasts and large mononuclear cells. At one day there was vascular congestion and marked edema, with separation of the liver cords. At two days there was decrease in the degree of the edema, and only a small degree of edema remained at seven days. PMN infiltration was greatly reduced at the third and seventh days. Congestion of the hepatic vessels, and to a lesser extent the sinusoids, was observed from the 12th hour to the seventh day.

After 30,000 rads, with study for 20 days, the findings in 43 rabbits studied at various intervals were characterized by vascular congestion and edema. The edema was present immediately after irradiation and gradually increased in intensity so that by the third day it was so marked and caused such an increase in volume of the extracellular space that there was considerable compression of the hepatic cells. There was a lesser degree of edema at 7 days, but congestion of the smaller vessels and some sinuosids persisted. Polymorphonuclear leukocyte infiltration was present immediately after irradiation, increased at 12 hours, remained constant to the second day, and was not prominent at three and seven days. Necrotic patches of the liver parenchyma were observed at two days. At seven days, sections of liver varied from apparently normal to marked and widespread destruction of the liver parenchyma. At 20 days, there was no evidence of hepatic cell damage.

After 50,000 rads, with study for one week, severe vascular congestion and periportal acute inflammatory cell reactions were observed immediately after irradiation, and at two and three days there were patchy necrotic areas diffusely distributed throughout the irradiated areas. Large areas of necrotic liver parenchyma were surrounded by groups or layers of viable, normal-appearing liver cells. In the degenerative areas, blood vessels were fragmented and surrounded by serum and erythrocytes in large quantities. The bile duct epithelium was swollen and often there were polymorphonuclear cells among the biliary epithelial cells or mixed with debris within the bile duct. By the seventh day there was complete destruction of the liver parenchyma in the irradiated zone, with no definite abnormality in the nonirradiated areas.

After 100,000 rads, with study for 2 ½ days, immediately after irradiation the liver cells were pale staining, there was some disorganization of hepatic cords, and there was marked vascular congestion and infiltration of polymorphonuclear leukocytes. At 1 ½ and 2 ½ days there were numerous small and large necrotic areas throughout the irradiated region, with many of the large areas showing evidence of complete destruction of the liver structure. These lesions were more extensive than those observed after 50,000 rads.

These observations of Ariel support the contention that hepatic cells are relatively resistant to the direct destructive actions of ionizing radiation. Furthermore, the early vascular congestion and edema in irradiated and nonirradiated areas and the inflammatory cell infiltration and portal fibrosis in irradiated areas at dose levels and sometimes at periods not associated with hepatic necrosis, together with the sharply defined patchy character of the necrosis when it did occur, tend to support strongly the prime role of damage to the fine vasculature and connective tissue in the pathogenesis of radiation-induced hepatic necrosis and fibrosis. This does not preclude a contributory role of direct injury to hepatic cells.

The induction of regeneration in the liver after irradiation by such means as partial hepatectomy or poisoning with carbon tetrachloride has been used to unmask hidden radiation injuries in liver cells, particularly nuclear injuries which become manifest in mitosis. Weinbren et al.[223,224] irradiated the two anterior liver lobes of rats with a single dose of 5000 rads, and after one day, one month, two months, and three months did a biopsy of the previously irradiated lobes and ligated the afferent vessels and duct of the previously shielded posterior lobes to produce infarct. The rats were then killed in groups at intervals of 29, 48, and 72 hr. In addition, groups of irradiated and control rats were kept for a year before the posterior lobes were infarcted, and the animals were killed 48 hr later.

The incidence of mitoses after infarction was affected only temporarily by previous irradiation, with complete inhibition lasting for only the first few days. After two months, the incidence in irradiated tissue was not significantly different from that in controls. Biopsy specimens taken from irradiated or nonirradiated livers at the time of the second operation (for ligation) could not be distinguished from one another microscopically. After regeneration had been stimulated by infarction, however, the differences between irradiated and control tissues were distinct and constant. Degenerate cells, mitotic abnormalities, and wide variations in nuclear size were the main distinctive features in the irradiated tissues. The appearance of the degenerate cells, together with its clear time relationship to the incidence of mitosis, strongly suggested that the degenerate cells became degenerate or necrotic in preparation for or during the process of mitosis.

Abnormal mitotic figures were high in incidence with respect to the total number of

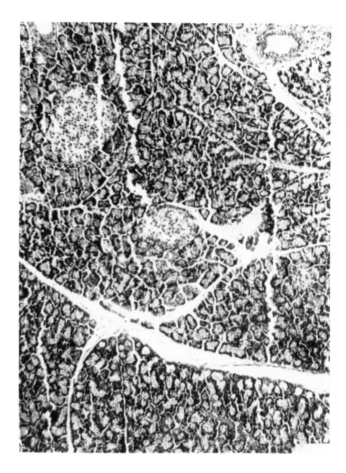

FIGURE 3.    Sections of normal rat pancreas. A. Section (approximately 200×) showing two islets of Langerhans in the midst of a mass of acinous tissue.

mitoses when hyperplasia was stimulated in liver tissues one month to one year after irradiation, with no significant reduction in the incidence of abnormalities with time. However, the incidence of the various types of mitotic aberrations was different after different periods of time, with anaphase bridges developing most frequently when the interval between irradiation and induced regeneration was relatively short, and with structural (chromosomal) changes predominating at longer intervals.

These authors found it difficult to ascribe this increased incidence of chromosome breakage to any particular factor, but noted that the progressive vascular changes, which are often caused by irradiation, may be associated with this type of mitotic abnormality, and that the factors associated with progressive atrophy of the liver might be related to the mitotic abnormalities. The different types of mitotic abnormality in the liver appeared to be directly related to the time interval between irradiation and mitosis, and not to the dividing or nondividing condition of cells at the time of irradiation.

## C. The Pancreas

Essentially, the pancreas contains two glands, an exocrine gland and an endocrine gland (Figure 3A). The exocrine component, which is the largest part, is a typical purely serous gland (Figure 3B) that secretes from one type of cell, cytologically, a

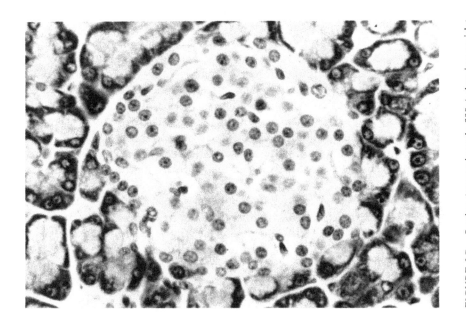

FIGURE 3C. Section (approximately 800×) showing an islet of Langerhans (center) surrounded by acini. (H. and E. stains.)

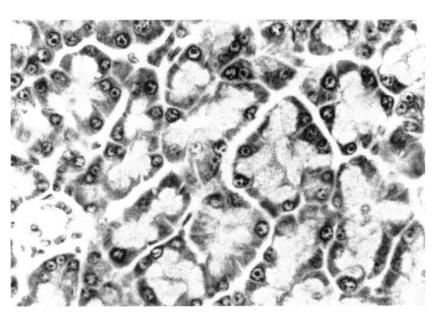

FIGURE 3B. Section (approximately 800×) showing acini, with a small duct (upper left).

digestive juice containing several digestive proenzymes which give rise to trypsin, amylase, lipase, and an enzyme like rennin. The secretion of this juice is stimulated by a hormone (secretin) formed in the duodenal mucosa, or it can be induced more directly via the vagus nerve supply. The pancreatic duct system drains into the duodenum via a main excretory duct. The endocrine component consists of diffusely scattered small islands (Islets of Langerhans) of epithelial cells (Figure 3C), an alcoholic extract of which is insulin, a hormone that regulates carbohydrate metabolism.

The exocrine glandular parenchyma is in the form of a compound tubuloalveolar gland containing purely serous alveoli. Each alveolus has a basement membrane of reticular fibers on which rests a single layer of pyramidal serous gland cells. In addition to these cells, central alveolar cells are present within alveoli. These central alveolar cells are duct cells, i.e., cells at the beginning of ducts surrounded by alveoli. The gland cells of a pancreatic alveolus usually do not become directly continuous with an intercalated duct in the way that more typical exocrine glands do. There are small secretory capillaries between the serous gland cells. Typical secretory ducts are lacking in the pancreas, but intercalated ducts are well developed and lined by a simple layer of flat or cuboidal epithelial cells. The excretory ducts are lined by a single layer of columnar epithelial cells.

The endocrine glandular parenchyma of the pancreas consists of many irregularly distributed Islets of Langerhans, which are small (ranging from the size of a few cells to a few mm) masses of epithelial cells infiltrated by labyrinths of capillaries. The Islet tissue consists of irregular and astamosing cords of epithelial cells separated by closely associated blood capillaries. By means of special techniques for demonstrating distinctive cytoplasmic granules, several cell types can be distinguished in the Islets on the basis of staining characteristics, solubility, etc.. These cells include alpha cells, which are fairly numerous in most Islets and contain water soluble granules; beta or B cells, which are smaller and much more numerous and contain alcohol soluble granules associated with insulin; and delta or D cells, which are rare.

The epithelial cells of the exocrine alveoli and of the Islets of Langerhans behave as longlived reverting postmitotic cells, i.e., they divide infrequently but are capable of proliferating upon demand. Both of these cell types are relatively resistant to the direct destructive actions of radiation. The pancreas is able to regenerate a few alveoli and even whole Islets after injury. Regeneration may follow duct ligation, which causes degeneration of alveoli alone, sparing the Islets, surgical excision or disease, with the regeneration stemming largely from proliferating duct tissue. Sometimes there are slender epithelial tubules or cords connecting ducts and Islets, which are remnants of tissue involved in the original development of the Islets. It is claimed that such tissue can regenerate Islets and perhaps alveoli also.

There has been relatively little experimental investigation of the pathologic effects of radiation on pancreas, and it has not been of a definitive nature or sufficient to indicate dose response relationships or provide histopathologic sequences of events.

Spaulding and Lusbaugh[230] studied the pancreatic Islets of monkeys and rats after massive doses of radiation delivered rapidly from a telesource of radiolanthinum. They found pyknosis and necrosis of the islet beta cells of monkeys that died within 200 hr after doses of 10,000 to 50,000 rads whole-body irradiation. Necrosis of the islet cells in rats was evident in 8 hr after doses of 2500 to 5000 rads. The alpha cells were more sensitive (LD50 about 5000 rads) than the beta cells (LD50 about 20,000 rads). The acinous cells showed no demonstrable morphologic change within the same time periods.

It is obvious that much more investigation is needed to establish more precisely the position of the pancreas and its component parts in the scale of radiosensitivity of tissues and to reveal the sequences of changes in the component parts of the pancreas at various times after irradiation.

It is clear, however, that substantial radiation-induced vascular damage may progress to sclerosis and obliteration of lumens of small arteries sufficient to cause marked secondary degeneration and loss of pancreatic epithelium, especially the acinous epithelium, long after irradiation with large doses (Figures 4A and 4B).

## II. MAJOR ENDOCRINE GLANDS

The gonads will be discussed in the following chapter.

In general, because the parenchymal cells of the mature pituitary, thyroid, parathyroid, and adrenal glands are reverting postmitotic cells and relatively resistant to the direct cytocidal actions of radiation, the early and late lesions caused by radiation in these glands are largely the result of damage to the fine vasculature and connective tissue responses, with impairment of circulation and secondary degeneration of dependent parenchymal cells. The sinusoidal phagocyte-lined vasculature of some of the endocrine glands (pituitary and adrenals) might conceivably contribute further to the low susceptibility of these organs to late effects of irradiation.

The interpretation of the direct effects of radiation on the endocrine glands is made difficult by the complex functional interrelationships of these glands among themselves and with other organs and tissues. A careful distinction must be made between those changes in gland cells that reflect functional responses to changes in other glands and tissues and those changes in gland cells that are the results of radiation damage to the cells. Therefore the radiation effects on endocrine glands are best observed, although not perfectly so, under conditions of localized irradiation of the individual glands. Unfortunately, there is relatively little of this sort of information.

The radiation histopathology of the endocrine tissue in the pancreas (Islets of Langerhans) and in the gonads is discussed in other parts of this book dealing specifically with these tissues or organs.

### A. The Pituitary Gland (Hypophysis)

The pituitary gland, or hypophysis, consists of the adenohypophysis and the neurohypophysis. The adenohypophysis includes the anterior lobe (pars distalis), an intermediate part (pars intermedia), and a tuberal part (pars tuberalis), while the neurohypophysis includes the median eminence, the infundibular stalk or stem, and the infundibular process.

The parenchymal or gland cells of the anterior lobe are arranged irregularly in cords and masses, and sometimes in small acinous-like structures, that are closely related to the sinusoids and are supported by reticular fibers. The sinusoids anastomose freely and are lined by phagocytic endothelium like that of the sinusoids of the adrenal cortex, liver, and spleen. Gland cells include chromophile cells and chromophobe cells, according to whether or not they become stained with dyes in certain histologic staining procedures. The chromophile cells are further distinguished with respect to the staining reactions of their specific granules when treated with the hematoxylin and eosin stains, namely, as acidophile cells (alpha cells) or as basophile cells (beta cells). The chromophobe cells are also called C cells (chief cells). The basophiles (beta cells) are the least numerous of these cells in man. The relative proportions of the three cell types are markedly variable.

These gland cells behave as reverting postmitotic cells and do not divide under normal conditions in the mature gland. Since mitoses are rarely observed in these cells, the observed changes in the proportions of the different cell types have been ascribed

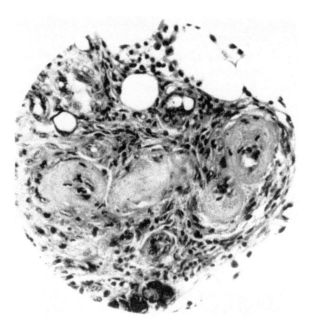

FIGURE 4.    Sections of rat pancreas 14 months after irradiation. A. Section (approximately 400×) showing markedly sclerotic small blood vessels with obliterated or partially obliterated lumens, surrounded by fibrotic tissue which has replaced
most of the acinous parenchyma.

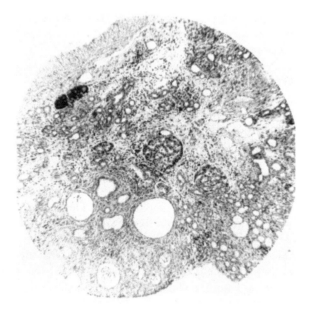

FIGURE 4B.    Section (approximately 100×) showing virtually
extreme artophy of the acinous parenchyma secondary to vascular damage, with two surviving but degenerating islets. (H.
and E. stains.) (From Casarett, G. W., *Radiat. Res. Suppl.*, 5,
246, 1964. With permission.)

to the transformation of one cell type to another. One of the most widely accepted concepts is that the chromophobes are relatively undifferentiated cells which can form granules and differentiate into one or another of the chromophilic types, and that this process may be reversible under certain conditions.

The hormones as secreted by the anterior lobe, and the cells that probably secrete them, include:

1. Somatotrophic hormone (STH), secreted by acidophile cells, more specifically a subclass called orangeophiles;
2. Follicle stimulating hormone (FSH), leutinizing hormone (LH) and prolactin, which form the gonadotropic hormone complex and are secreted by basal cells, more specifically by a subclass called the delta basophiles;
3. Thyrotropic hormone (TSH), secreted by basophile cells, more specifically by a subclass called beta basophiles;
4. Adrenocorticotropic hormone (ACTH), the cellular origin of which is not definitely known.

The pars intermedia contains basophile cells, which extend into the neural lobe, and chromophobe cells. The abundant capillaries of this part are continuous with the capillary bed of the neural lobe and with the sinusoids of the anterior lobe. The pars intermedia secretes under neural control a hormone called intermedin, which causes expression of melanocytes and darkening of the skin. The pars tuberalis contains cords of cuboidal columnar cells of no known hormonal function and some acidophile and basophile cells.

The neurohypophysis consists largely of nonmyelinated nerves of the hypothalamo-hypophysial tract enclosed in a protoplasmic sheath by cells called pituicytes, but in the posterior lobe the nerve fibers and the pituicytes become disassociated and run parallel courses, each ending with processes on pericapillary connective tissue. It is believed that the neurohypophysial granules called Herring bodies represent neurosecretory material formed in the cells of the supraoptic and periventricular nuclei, transported along the nerve fibers and stored at nerve terminals in the infundibular process. The neurohypophysial hormones include oxytocin which causes contraction of the smooth muscle of the uterus, and vasopressin which raises blood pressure by causing contraction of the smooth muscle in small blood vessels and which also performs an antidiuretic action by promoting reabsorption of water in the kidney (mainly in the thin segment of the loop of Henle).

The epithelial cells of the hypophysis are reverting postmitotic cells and are relatively resistant to the direct destructive actions of radiation. The neural elements of the hypophysis are highly radioresistant.

Long-term follow-up studies of weanling (28-day old) male rats that had been giving single localized pituitary doses of high energy deuteron particles were performed by Tobias et al.[238] and Van Dyke et al.[239] In the first of these studies, doses from 3,000 to 25,000 reps (Roentgen equivalents physical) were given, and the observations on groups of rats sacrificed at intervals of four days to nine months after irradiation led to the following conclusions:

1. The degree of destruction of the pituitary depends on both dose and postirradiation time;
2. Prompt and complete destruction of the pituitary was caused only by doses of 18,900 reps or larger, and after doses of 6,300 reps or less the destruction was not complete nine months after irradiation;

3.  There was no evidence of stimulation of the pituitary in terms of morphology or function;
4.  There was no recovery of the pituitary from the radiation damage;
5.  No difference in sensitivity among pituitary cell types was seen;
6.  Doses from 6,300 to 18,900 reps impaired increases in body weight and thyroid weight soon, but degeneration of testes occurred much later.

The long-term study by VanDyke et al.[239] of immature male rats receiving pituitary irradiation was an extension of the previous study by Tobias et al., including smaller doses of deuteron radiation (945 to 6300 reps) and longer postirradiation study (3 to 27 months). The endocrine changes depended on both dose and increasing time after irradiation. The time taken to reach the maximal effect varied inversely with the size of the dose. The effects on pituitary structures included decrease in size of all lobes, loss of demarcation between lobes, increased connective tissue in the surrounding membrane and supporting framework, and frequent small hemorrhages.

Degranulation and disappearance of acidophile cells of the anterior lobe occurred soonest and at the lowest dose level, with lesser degrees of such changes in basophiles.

Van Dyke et al. considered the degranulation and disappearance of chromophiles and the vacuolation of basophiles (resembling the vacuolation after castration or thyroidectomy) as degenerative changes and as radiation damage. Since the numbers and proportions of acidophiles, basophiles, and chromophobes were not determined or given in the report, it is difficult to assess the extent to which these reported changes were indirect functional effects of hormonal changes causing transformation of chromophile cells to chromophobe cells, or basophile cells to castration cells or thyroidectomy cells, and the extent to which the reported changes were the direct or indirect degenerative effects of irradiation on the gland cells themselves.

In this study the changes in other organs that are dependent on the pituitary hormones were observed to appear in the following order: reduction of adrenal weight with atrophy of adrenal cortex; decrease in size and activity of the thyroid; atrophy of testes; and regression of male accessory organs.

Simpson et al.[237] extended the studies of effects of deuteron beam irradiation of the pituitary to immature monkeys (8 to 15 months old) given 4500 or 9000 reps in a single dose and necropsied about 28 to 52 months later. The irradiated pituitaries were reduced in size, in all lobes. The general pattern of histologic structure was usually still distinguishable, and the normal distribution of specific cell types was usually maintained. All lobes, especially the intermediate lobe, showed regions of extensive cell destruction or widespread vacuolation of parenchymal cells. The walls of the blood vessels were often thickened. The authors concluded that the reduced size and partial degranulation which frequently characterized the irradiated glands may have been secondary to reduced vascularity resulting from vascular sclerosis. Scar tissue replaced parenchyma where small localized hemorrhages had occurred secondary to blood vessel damage.

## B. The Adrenal Glands

The cortex of the adrenal gland is composed of three layers, namely, from outside inward, the thin zona glomerulosa under the capsule, the thick middle zone or zona fasciculata, and the moderately thick inner zone or zona reticularis which surrounds the medulla (Figures 5A and 5B).

The adrenal cortex is involved in the maintenance of water and electrolyte balance, carbohydrate balance, and the connective tissue of the body. The disturbances of body function caused by cortical deficiency are reversed by treatment with various cortical

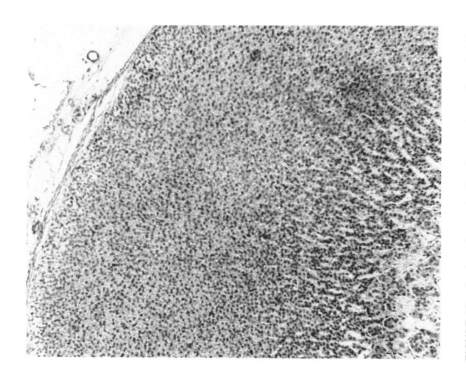

FIGURE 5B. Section of normal adrenal cortex (approximately 200×) showing the thin zona glomerulosa beneath the capsule, the intermediate zone (fasciculata) and the inner zone (reticularis).

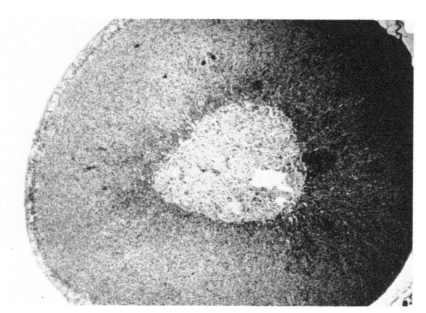

FIGURE 5. Sections of rat adrenal glands. A. Section of normal adrenal (approximately 50×) showing the thick cortex and the central medulla.

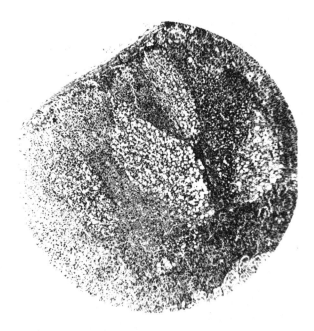

FIGURE 5C.   Section (approximately 100×) a year after irradiation showing marked vacuolation (fatty metamorphosis)
and hyperplasia of the cortex. (H. and E. stains.) (C from Casarett, G. W., U.S. Atomic Energy Commission Report UR-
201, Washington, 1952.)

extracts (or through synthetic products), such as the mineralocorticoids (deoxycorti-
costerone and aldosterone) which influence water and electrolyte balance, and the glu-
cocorticoids (cortisone and hydrocortisone) which influence the metabolism of carbohydrate, fat, and protein.

The extent to which different zones of the cortex serve different or the same functions is not entirely clear. The impression has been gained that the zona glomerulosa
is more involved than the other zones in the production of a deoxycorticosterone-like
compound, and that cortisone may be secreted more by the zona fasciculata.

In addition to specific zonal responses in the cortex to various specific types of imbalances in the body, the adrenal cortex seems to respond with hyperfunction in a
nonspecific fashion to many different kinds of stresses. The morphologic response is
generally similar to that which can be caused by the administration of certain doses of
adrenocorticotropic hormone and is mediated through the pituitary. There is hypertrophy and hyperplasia of the cortex, and there may be an increase in cortical lipid (Figure
5C) which may be followed in later stages of stress by a decrease in lipid droplets below
normal levels. The cholesterol and ascorbic acid content of the cortex may also be
reduced during stress. Control of the adrenocortical activities seems to be mediated
largely by the anterior lobe of the pituitary gland through its secretion of the adrenocorticotropic hormone. There also appears to be some functional relation between the
adrenal cortex and the sex glands.

The parenchymal cells of the adrenal cortex and medulla are reverting postmitotic
cells and are relatively resistant to the direct cytocidal actions of radiation. The medullary cells secrete the hormones epinephrine and norepinephrine.

Some of the morphologic changes which may be observed in the adrenal glands after
irradiation of the entire body or parts of the body, even if the adrenals are not irradiated, are changes related to the nonspecific response of the adrenals (mediated by the

pituitary) to stresses, among which may be included radiation damage to tissues. Among the early adrenal changes of this kind are rapid decreases in the amount of adrenal cortical lipids, adrenal cholesterol, and ascorbic acid associated with an increased secretion of adrenocortical hormones (steroids). Later there may be adrenal cortical hypertrophy and increase in cortical lipid. The later hypertrophic changes in the adrenals are the result of persistent stress or functional demands for adrenal hormones (Figure 5C).

Although the parenchymal cells of the mature adrenal gland are generally long-lived reverting postmitotic cells and relatively radioresistant, the susceptibility of the nonirradiated adrenal cortical zones to congestion, hemorrhages, and destruction of small numbers of cells, associated with episodes of acute functional demand, results more or less frequently in the presence of small numbers of mitotic cells which are more radiosensitive. Aside from the functional responses of the gland to stress, the pathogenesis of early radiation-induced degenerative changes in the adrenals involves primarily radiation damage to the fine vasculature and impairment of circulation, with engorgement of the small nutrient blood vessels and sinusoids, increased capillary and sinusoidal permeability, interstitial edema, hemorrhages, and secondary degeneration (pyknosis, vacuolization) of the parenchymal cells.

The degree of these early changes is directly dose-dependent. With doses of moderate size the early changes may be transient and resolve rapidly, with substantial recovery of the circulation, subsidence of the edema, regeneration of lost parenchymal cells, and repair of hemorrhagic regions. However, the vascular disruption and circulatory impairment following large doses may be so severe and persistent as to cause areas of destruction and necrosis of parenchyma and to prevent substantial regeneration of parenchymal cells from those cells which survive. Under these circumstances repair by secondary intention occurs in the form of proliferation of connective tissue and scar formation. It should be emphasized that, as is the case with other endocrine glands, the adrenals may undergo a delayed phase of parenchymal degeneration secondary to the slowly progressive deterioration of the fine vasculature and circulation and the progressive interstitial fibrosis, even after substantial recovery from the initial degenerative phase, and that the postirradiation time necessary to reach this second phase of parenchymal degeneration is inversely related to the size of the dose.

Englestad and Torgersen[241] showed that a dose of 1000 R or less does not induce demonstrable changes in rabbit adrenals. After 1500 R in a single dose, only mild changes occur. At 1700 R, significant changes in the adrenals result. After doses between 2000 and 2500 R, cortical degeneration, inflammation, and severe hyperemia occur. After 3000 R there is progressive cortical fibroatrophy.

## C. The Thyroid Gland

The thyroid parenchyma is arranged in the form of spherical follicles of varying size, lined by a layer of simple epithelium (reverting postmitotic cells) and containing variable amounts of colloid (Figures 6A and 6B). The follicles are intimately enclosed by richly anastomosing baskets of capillaries. Between the capillary beds and adjacent follicles are meshes of lymphatic capillaries. The follicular colloid is an active reservoir containing noniodinated and iodinated protein in various proportions, thyroglobulin (thyroxin, diodothyronine, and triiodothyronine bound to a globulin), and also some mucoproteins and enzymes (a proteolytic enzyme, peroxidase, and a mucinase).

The uptake of iodine from the blood by the thyroid gland, the conversion of iodine to the active hormonal principle of the gland, and the release of thyroid hormone into the circulation are affected by the thyrotropic hormone of the pituitary gland. An excess or a reduction of thyroid hormone in the blood inhibits or stimulates, respec-

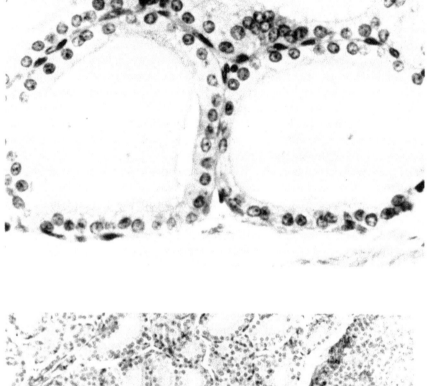

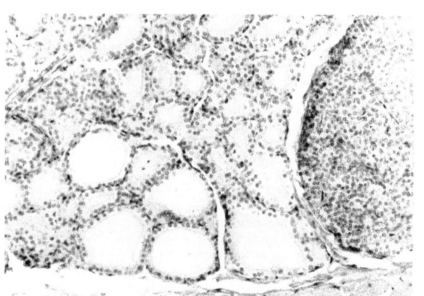

FIGURE 6B.   Section (approximately 800×) showing normal colloid-filled thyroid follicles lined by a single layer of cuboidal epithelial cells. (H. and E. stains.)

FIGURE 6.   Sections of normal rat thyroid and parathyroid glands. A. Section (approximately 200×) showing normal thyroid follicles filled with colloid (above) and normal parathyroid gland (below).

tively, the secretion of the pituitary thyrotropic hormone, resulting in reduction or increase, respectively, of thyroid activity. Since the primary effect of thyroid hormone is on the basal metabolic rate, it influences metabolism and growth in general. The reverting postmitotic epithelial parenchymal cells of the thyroid are relatively resistant to the direct destructive actions of ionizing radiations.

Because of the relative resistance of the thyroid epithelial cells to the direct cytocidal actions of radiation, early severe radionecrosis, which requires massive doses for its production, is caused largely by severe damage to the fine vasculature and associated acute inflammatory, edematous, and hemorrhagic consequences, with impairment of the circulation. The delayed radionecrosis or atrophy following more moderate doses is largely secondary to a more slowly progressive degeneration and obliteration of the fine vasculature and impairment of circulation. Under these circumstances the degree of secondary parenchymal damage (atrophy) is directly dependent upon dose for a given time after irradiation, and is also directly dependent upon time after irradiation.

The earliest histopathologic effects of radiation on the normal mature thyroid gland are those related to damage to capillaries and to the endothelium of other small blood vessels and which give rise within hours or days to circulatory congestion and increased capillary permeability, with interstitial edema of the stroma and some interstitial infiltration of leukocytes. Similar changes in the endothelium of arterioles may result in subendothelial edema of the vessel wall. With large doses the damage to the fine vasculature may be severe enough to cause multiple small hemorrhages interstitially and even intrafollicularly, as well as more prolonged and severe acute edematous and inflammatory changes. This acute inflammatory response, where severe, may cause localized vacuolar degeneration of epithelial cells or focal sloughing of follicular cells into the follicular lumens, with subsequent degeneration of the cells. These early changes in the thyroid follicular epithelium are variable in degree and distribution in the gland, in relation to the variability of the degree of distribution of the acute edematous, inflammatory, and extravasational or hemorrhagic events. The colloid content of follicles becomes reduced, especially in follicles showing greater degrees of degeneration or sloughing of epithelium, and phagocytes may enter the follicles and ingest colloid. The rupture of follicular basement membranes, the degeneration and sloughing of follicular epithelium, the loss of follicular colloid, and hypoplasia and atrophy of the gland (secondary to the acute inflammatory changes) may continue progressively for a time until the acute inflammation has subsided and adequate microcirculation is restored.

After moderate radiation doses, the regeneration of follicular epithelium following the resolution of the early acute inflammatory changes may be rapid and fairly complete, and there may remain only subtle residual damage in the fine vasculature and interfollicular stroma. The greater vascular damage and acute inflammatory changes caused by larger doses result in greater degrees of epithelial degeneration and less complete regeneration, with more obvious residual damage in the vasculature and stroma.

After the regenerative phase there is slowly progressive degeneration of arterioles, capillaries, and venules, with eventual spotty narrowing or obliteration of lumens and increases in the amount and density of perivascular and interstitial connective tissue (Figure 7A). The rate of these progressive changes in the fine vessels and connective tissue varies directly with the size of the dose and the degree of initial damage. These changes eventually result in a second and progressive phase of degeneration and loss of follicular epithelium and follicles secondary to impairment of circulation (Figures 7B and 7C). The postirradiation time of occurrence for a given degree of such delayed parenchymal damage varies inversely with the size of the dose and the rate of progression of the vascular degeneration. In regions of less affected vasculature and connec-

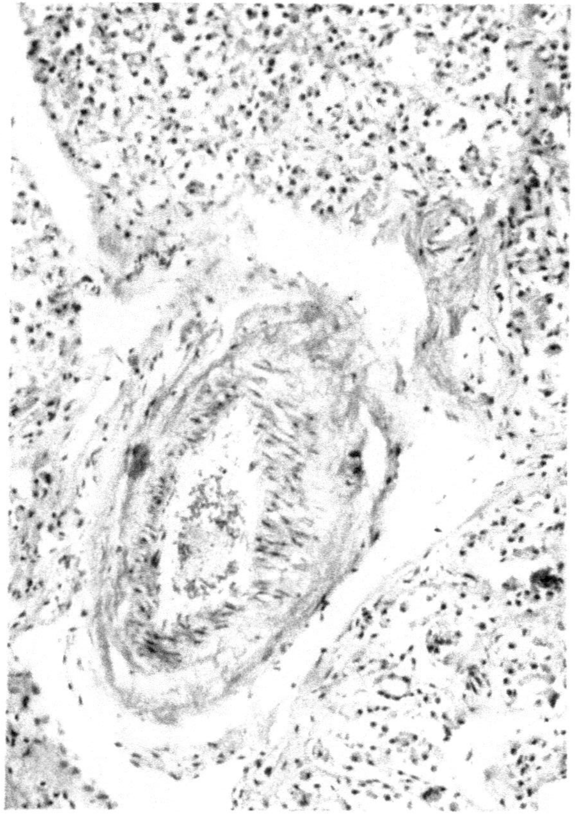

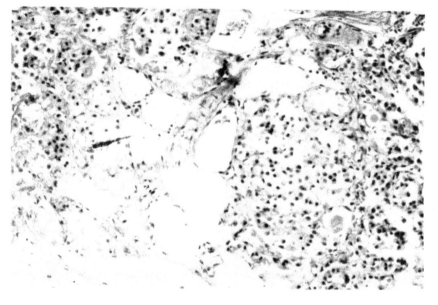

FIGURE 7B.    Degeneration, sloughing, and loss of follicular epithelium, loss of follicular colloid, and arteriolosclerosis.

FIGURE 7.    Sections of nodular atrophic thyroid glands from dogs about three years after 1820R X-irradiation. A. Perivascular and medial fibrosis of large vessel (central), lymphatic dilatation around large vessel, sclerosis of arteriolar walls, loss of follicular colloid, and degeneration and sloughing of follicular epithelium.

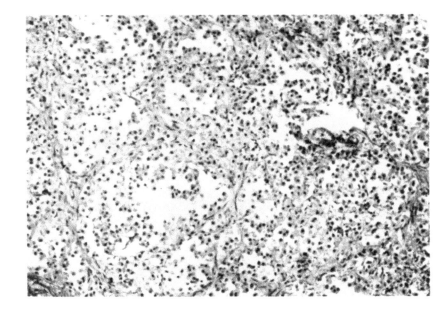

FIGURE 7D. Nodule containing enlarged follicles with hyperplastic epithelium, but without colloid. (H. and E. stains; magnification approximately 200×.) (From Michaelson, S., Quinlan, W., Casarett, G. W., and Mason, W. B., *Radiat. Res.*, 30, 38, 1967. With permission.)

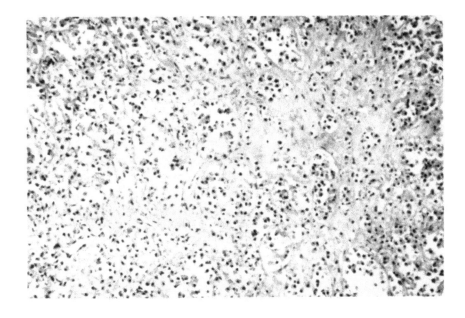

FIGURE 7C. Follicular epithelial degeneration, follicular atrophy, and loss of colloid associated with interstitial fibrosis.

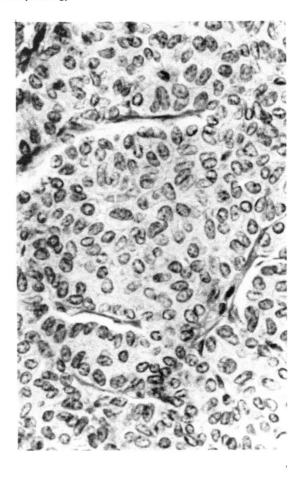

FIGURE 8.    Sections of rat parathyroid glands. A. Section
(approximately 800×) of normal parathyroid.

tive tissue, and less affected follicles, the follicular cells show compensatory cellular
hyperplasia (Figure 7D).

Michaelson et al.[254] have demonstrated the development of delayed radiation-induced primary hypothyroidism in adult dogs about two to four years after X-ray doses
ranging from 1000 to 2100 R. The lower the dose the later the hypothyroidism appeared. The pathogenesis of the thyroid changes associated with the development of
this hypothyroidism appeared to involve primarily the slowly progressive and patchy
degeneration and fibrosis of the fine vasculature and interfollicular stroma, with eventual secondary degeneration of the follicular epithelium and follicles in some regions,
with hyperplastic reactions in less effected regions, and with the production of atrophic
but nodular thyroid glands containing little colloid (Figure 7).

## D. The Parathyroid Gland

The parenchyma of the parathyroid gland (Figures 6A and 8A) consists of dense
cords or masses of gland cells of two general types: the principal cells, which are the
most numerous, and the oxyphile cells, which are characterized by the eosinophilic
granulation and larger size. There is a rich capillary network between cords or masses
of gland cells. The parathyroid hormone is involved in the homeostatic regulation of
the calcium ion concentration in the body fluids. There is an increased secretion of
the hormone in response to a lowered plasma concentration of calcium, which in turn

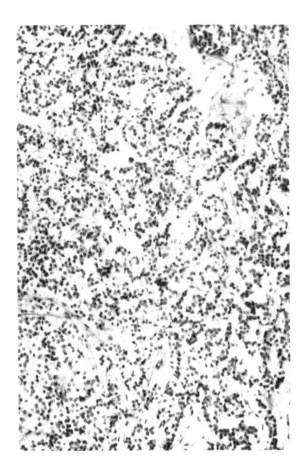

FIGURE 8B. Section (approximately 200×) of parathyroid about six months after 2000R, showing degeneration of many cells, with considerable disorganization of parenchymal architecture, associated with arteriolosclerosis and interstitial fibrosis. (H. and E. stains.)

causes an increased dissolution of bone mineral through increased osteoclastic resorption of bone. The parenchymal cells of the parathyroid glands are reverting postmitotic cells and are relatively resistant to the direct cytocidal actions of radiation.

The histopathologic effects of localized irradiation of the parathyroid glands have not been studied sufficiently to reveal the sequence of events after various doses of radiation. However, on the basis of many incidental observations it does appear that the parenchymal cells are relatively radioresistant, as are the parenchymal cells of the pituitary, thyroid, and adrenal gland, and similarly may show early degenerative changes secondary to acute edematous and inflammatory changes caused by radiation damage to the fine vasculature, or more delayed postrecovery degeneration secondary to the progressive deterioration of the fine vasculature and interstitial fibrosis (Figure 8B). Doses of radiation from external sources sufficiently large to cause atrophy of the thyroid gland may cause atrophy of the irradiated parathyroid glands also.

Chapter 5

# THE GONADS

## I. THE TESTES

The testes are compound tubular glands divided into intercommunicating lobules which contain convoluted seminiferous tubules (Figure 1A). In the normal sexually mature male, the convoluted seminiferous tubules are lined by complex stratified seminiferous epithelium composed of the sustentacular (nutrient and supporting) cells of Sertoli and the much more numerous spermatogenic cells which undergo proliferation and transformation to form mature spermatozoa (Figure 1B).

The interstitial (intertubular) tissue outside the basement membranes of seminiferous tubules contains thin collagenous fibers, small blood and lymph vessels, nerves, fibroblasts, embryonic perivascular mesenchymal cells, macrophages, mast cells, and the specific interstitial cells of Leydig to which has been ascribed the production of the male sex hormone testosterone.

In general, in seminiferous tubules actively engaged in spermatogenesis, the Sertoli cells are attached to the basement membrane and separated from one another by crowded primitive spermatogenic cells, the spermatogonia. In general, the more primitive stages of the spermatogenic cells are located near the basement membrane of the tubule and the more differentiated stages are found closer to the lumen of the tubule, Spermatogenesis starts with primitive type A spermatogonia, which proliferate mitotically to reproduce themselves and to produce differentiating Type A spermatogenia, intermediate spermatogonia, and type B spermatogonia along the inner surface of the basement membrane (Figure 2). Likewise, these differentiating spermatogonia undergo a series of mitotic divisions, with the production of primary spermatocytes which grow, leave the basement membrane, and move toward the lumen. During this period of growth, the nucleus of the primary spermatocyte undergoes a series of changes in preparation for the first of the two reduction or maturation (meiotic) divisions, by which spermatids containing a haploid number of chromosomes are produced. With full development, the primary spermatocyte divides into two smaller secondary spermatocytes, each of which soon divides to produce two smaller spermatids near the lumen. Spermatids then move toward the basement membrane, closer to Sertoli cells, and undergo a complex metamorphosis (spermiogenesis) to form mature spermia, which then move to the tubule lumen for passage through the duct system to the epididymis (Figure 1C) and ejaculatory ducts.

In general, a cross section of a seminiferous tubule reveals circumferentially the same combination of basic cell types and generations, division activities, and degrees of differentiation among the cell generations in the spermatogenic epithelium lining the tubule. However, in a longitudinal section of a tubule, the epithelium is changing continuously in the longitudinal direction, with respect to division activity and degrees of differentiation among the basic spermatogenic cell generations. Spermatogenesis proceeds in a wave-like manner along the length of the tubule.

In man, the "spermatogenic wave", i.e., time between the division of primitive Type A spermatogonial stem cells and the completion of the spermatid metamorphisis to spermatozoa and their extrusion into the tubule lumen (approximately four spermatogenic cycles) has been estimated to be approximately 64 days.[265] The spermatogenic wave tends to be shorter in small mammals, e.g., about 48 days for the rat.[25]

In addition to producing sperm cells, the testes, presumably through the production

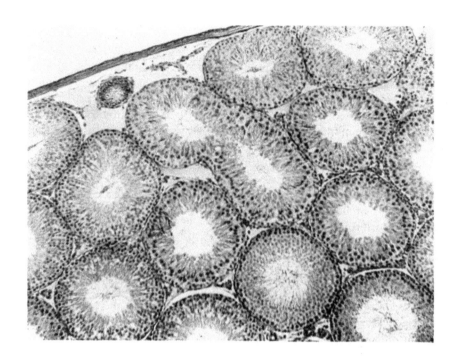

FIGURE 1B.   Section (approximately 200×) showing seminiferous tubules with their stratified spermatogenic epithelium and small amounts of intertubular tissue.

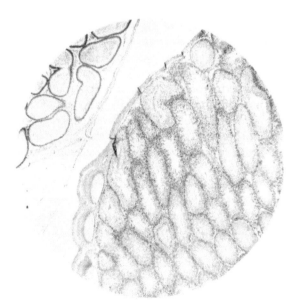

FIGURE 1A.   Sections of normal rat testis and epididymis. A. Section (approximately 50×) showing seminiferous tubules of testis (below) and tubules of the epididymis (above). (From Casarett, G. W., *Radiat. Res. Suppl.*, 5, 246, 1964. With permission.)

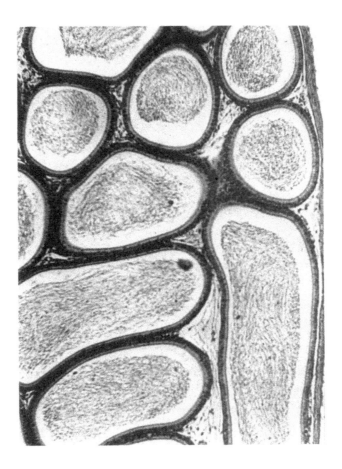

FIGURE 1C. Section (approximately 200×) showing epididymal tubules lined by a single layer of cuboidal epithelial cells and containing sperm. (H. and E. stains.)

of testosterone by interstitial Leydig cells, govern the development and maintain the secondary sexual organs and characteristics, including libido.

The sperm cells and spermatogenic cells of the seminiferous epithelium are sensitive to many different kinds of noxious factors, such as infectious disease and other pathologic conditions, dietary deficiencies, alcoholism, local injury or inflammation, conditions relating to mental depression, and even the normal temperature of the body. In most of these conditions the more mature spermatogenic cells seem more sensitive than the more primitive cells, although all may eventually be affected. Upon removal of the noxious influence, if some of the primitive spermatogonia have remained intact at the basement membrane, regeneration of the spermatogenic epithelium from these remaining stem cells may take place to varying degrees. In experimental animals sterilized temporarily by X-ray exposure, neoformation of primitive spermatogonia from mitotically dividing Sertoli cells or from transforming fibrocytes in or near the basement membrane or from interstitial mesenchymal cells penetrating the basement membrane, have been suggested on the basis of observation of transitional forms.[41,62]

In man, spermatogenesis continues well into the senescent period of life. However, from the middle of life there is generally an increasing involution or atrophy of individual tubules with increasing age.

On the basis of the direct cellular destructive action of ionizing radiation, most of the type A spermatogonia (vegetative and differentiating intermitotic cells), i.e., those

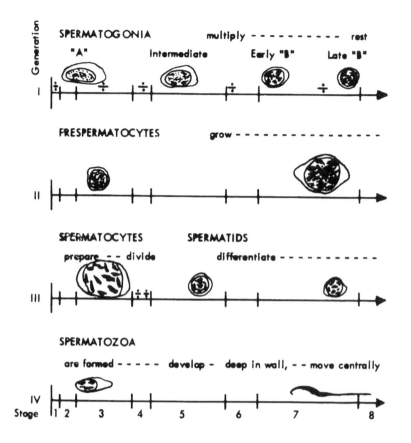

FIGURE 2.    Diagram of a cycle of the "spermatogenic wave" in the rat. (From Casarett, A. P. and Casarett, G. W., U.S. Atomic Energy Commission Reports UR-496 and 497. 1957.)

with relatively short intermitotic periods (within a few hours), are highly radiosensitive, the intermediate and type B spermatogonia (differentiating intermitotic cells) are only slightly less sensitive, spermatocytes (differentiating intermitotic cells) are somewhat less radiosensitive, and the spermatids and spermatozoa (fixed postmitotic cells) are relatively radioresistant. That fraction of the primitive Type A spermatogonia which have relatively long interphase periods (at least equal to the duration of a spermatogenic wave) and which appear to act as reserve (reverting postmitotic) cells until called upon to proliferate in the initiation of spermatogenic cycles, appear to be fairly radioresistant in the resting condition.

The simple epithelium lining the epididymis (reverting postmitotic cells) is relatively radioresistant. The Sertoli cells and Leydig cells (reverting postmitotic cells) are relatively radioresistant.

Aside from the still unresolved question of heterotypic formation of primitive type A spermatogonia from other types of cells, the fact that the relatively small numbers of type A spermatogonia with long intermitotic periods are more radioresistant than those with short intermitotic periods helps to explain the apparent survival of some irradiated type A spermatogonia, even after fairly large single doses of radiation. Much smaller single doses may temporarily reduce the population of type A spermatogonia almost as much.

The highly radiosensitive spermatogonia may be quickly reduced in numbers by a small amount after radiation doses as small as a few rads. Higher doses cause correspondingly greater decrease in numbers. The mechanisms by which radiation causes reduction in spermatogonia include: temporary inhibition of mitosis; reproductive sterilization of some of the cells; mitosis-linked cell necrosis; the normal process of maturation of spermatogonia into primary spermatocytes after completing their mitotic divisions; and, to some extent, the precocious maturation of spermatogonia into primary spermatocytes before completion of their usual number of mitotic divisions. The relative contributions of these various mechanisms to the reduction in numbers of spermatogonia may vary with the size of the radiation dose or with the dose rate or fractionation schedule. The degree of radiation effect on spermatogonia and spermatocytes depends also upon their stages of mitotic activity and differentiation in the spermatogenic cycle.

The more mature, more radioresistant spermatogenic cells may continue the normal process of maturation into sperm cells after irradiation. If the radiation dose has been large enough to markedly reduce the number of spermatogonia and to inhibit their regeneration for a substantial period of time, e.g., longer than the time required for spermatogenesis from type A spermatogonium to a mature sperm, there may develop a maturation depletion of spermatogenic cells, in the order of normal maturation, before regeneration of type A spermatogonia has been completed.

An additional mechanism contributing to the reduction in the number of sperm cells produced after irradiation is the radiation injury to spermatocytes. Although direct destruction of large numbers of primary spermatocytes may require relatively large doses, moderate doses are capable of injuring these cells to the extent that some of them may die in the attempt to divide or may produce fewer normal daughter cells. Direct destruction of spermatids or spermia requires much larger doses.

In general, then, moderate doses of radiation largely affect the spermatogonia, with first a decrease in their number and with older germ cell generations undergoing maturation and depletion and disappearing in the order in which they were formed, until a point of maximum hypoplasia is reached. The destruction of some of the cells of more mature generations by larger doses may hasten the process of depletion to some extent. The degree and duration of depletion of the spermatogenic epithelium are largely the result of the degree of depletion of spermatogonia, the length of time taken for the spermatogenic process, and the length of time during which there has been a reduction in number or cessation of replacement of the spermatogonia.

The bulk of pertinent experimental evidence indicates that the primary effects of irradiation on the spermatogenic epithelium are direct, in that irradiation of the body with the testes shielded does not produce them.[25] However, this does not preclude the possibility that irradiation of the rest of the body with doses large enough to cause serious illness could indirectly affect spermatogenesis, especially the more mature spermatogenic cells, e.g., through the production of nutritional deficiencies.

Most studies of sequences of radiation effects on spermatogenesis in mammals have been done on rodents, but the effects of radiation on the testes are qualitatively similar in all laboratory mammals studied and in man. They vary quantitatively according to differences among species in the radiosensitivity of the spermatogenic epithelium and the recovery capacity of the seminiferous epithelium. When permanence of sterilization is the point in question, the natural capacity for germ-cell regeneration in the species is as important as the radiosensitivity of spermatogenic cells.

With a single dose of X-rays large enough to nearly deplete the spermatogenic epithelium, but small enough to permit active spermatogonial regeneration before all mature spermia are removed from the seminiferous tubules (e.g., 325 rads to the rat testes), there is mitotic inhibition and necrosis of some spermatogonia in sensitive stages of spermatogenesis which lead to reduction of spermatogonial numbers in the

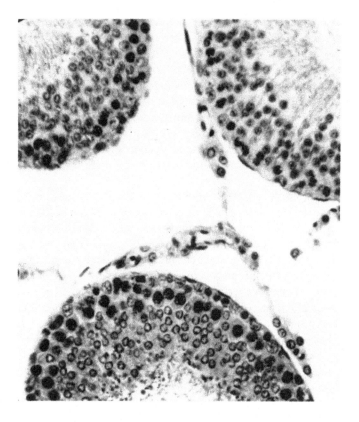

FIGURE 3.    Sections of rat testes after 325R of X-rays. A. Section (approximately 400×) four days after irradiation, showing degeneration of some spermatogonia and mild decrease in number of spermatogonia.

first few days after irradiation (Figure 3A). In addition, there are precocious differentiation of some spermatogonia, mitotic abnormalities in some spermatocytes (Figure 3B), and varying degrees of interstitial (intertubular) edema, with varying amounts of proteinacous material in the fluid. By the fourth day there has been considerable reduction in the number of spermatogonia in sections of tubules in some stages of spermatogenesis, but with little or no reduction in sections of tubules in other stages of spermatogenesis (Figure 3A). In some tubules there is evidence of abnormal divisions of primary spermatocytes in the form of unequal repartition of chromosomal material between daughter cells or abnormal numbers and sizes of nuclei (Figure 3B).

By the 11th day, there has been a further loss of spermatogonia, marked in some tubules and associated with the beginning of reduction of spermatocytes, but lesser in degree in sections of tubules in other stages of spermatogenesis (Figure 3C). By the 18th day, the reduction of spermatogonia is generally marked, and there is considerable reduction in the number of primary spermatocytes, varying in degree according to the stage of the spermatogenesis (Figure 3D). Small areas of intertubular edema may still be seen at this time. By the 25th day, there is still further maturation depletion of spermatogenic cells in some tubules, but small numbers of spermatogonia are regenerating in other tubules (Figure 4A). By the 32nd day after 325 rads, when spermatocytes and spermatids have largely disappeared and sperm cells have been reduced in number, spermatogonia are actively regenerating in some of the tubules (Figure 4B).

At about three to four weeks after larger single doses, e.g., 750 rad to rat testes, the seminiferous tubules are generally markedly depleted of spermatogenic cells, except

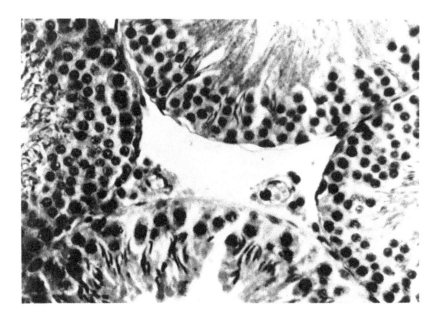

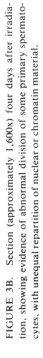

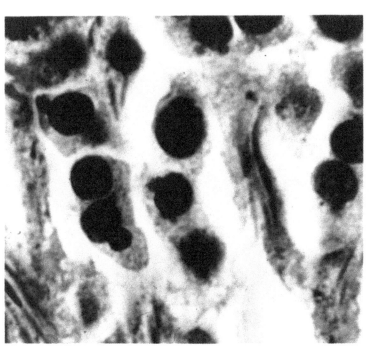

FIGURE 3C. Section (approximately 400×) 11 days after irradiation, showing more advanced loss of spermatogonia and considerable decrease in number of spermatocytes in the tubule at the left.

FIGURE 3B. Section (approximately 1,600x) four days after irradiation, showing evidence of abnormal division of some primary spermatocytes, with unequal repartition of nuclear or chromatin material.

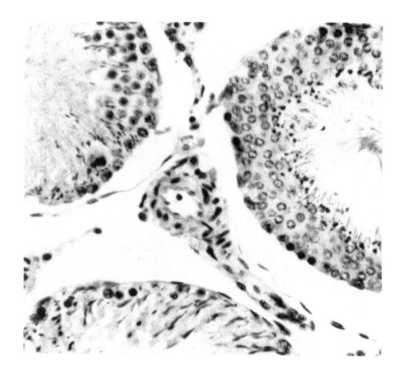

FIGURE 4. Sections of rat testes after X-irradiation. A. Section (approximately 400×) 25 days after 325R, showing marked maturation depletion of spermatogenic cells in one tubule (right) and less in the other tubules, according to spermatogenic stage, and regeneration of some spermatogonia in the upper tubule.

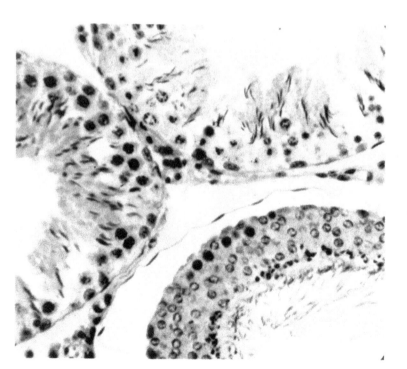

FIGURE 3D. Section (approximately 400×) 18 days after irradiation, showing marked decrease in number of spermatogonia and moderately marked loss of spermatocytes, variable among tubule sections according to stage of spermatogenesis, with evident necrosis of some spermatocytes. (H. and E. stains.) (From Casarett, A. P. and Casarett, G. W., U.S. Atomic Energy Commission Reports UR 496 and 497, 1957.)

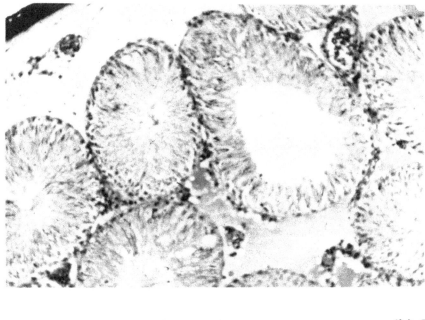

FIGURE 4C. Section (approximately 200×) 25 days after 750R, showing virtually complete maturation depletion of spermatogenic cells, except for developing sperm, and little regeneration of spermatogonia.

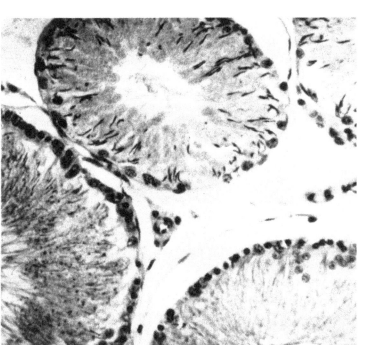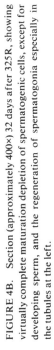

FIGURE 4B. Section (approximately 400×) 32 days after 325R, showing virtually complete maturation depletion of spermatogenic cells, except for developing sperm, and the regeneration of spermatogonia especially in the tubules at the left.

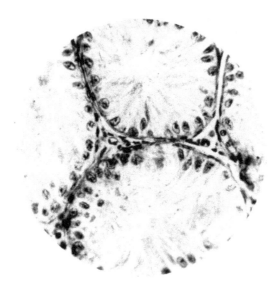

FIGURE 4D.   Section (approximately 400×) about 6 weeks
after a larger dose, showing virtually complete maturation depletion of spermatogenic epithelium, including sperm, with no
regeneration of spermatogonia and only Sertoli cell nuclei remaining along the basement membrane. (H. and E. stains.) (A
and B from Casarett, A. P. and Casarett, G. W., U.S. Atomic
Energy Commission Reports UR 496 and 497, 1957.)

for developing spermatozoa, and spermatogonial regeneration is more delayed (Figure
4C). Following still higher doses, e.g., 1500 rads or greater, to rat testes, depletion of
the spermatogenic epithelium tends to be extreme at about a month after irradiation,
leaving only Sertoli cells (Figure 4D). Regeneration of spermatogonia may be greatly
delayed, if it occurs at all, and recovery of the spermatogenic epithelium, when it does
occur, tends to be incomplete. Large doses may cause such extreme and prolonged
depletion of spermatogenic epithelium associated with such severe vascular damage
and subsequent vascular sclerosis that permanent atrophy of the seminiferous tubules
results. Under these conditions the tubules may eventually collapse and shrink into
compact masses, and the interstitial tissue may condense in space (Figure 5A and 5B).
There may also be eventual fatty infiltration and fibrosis of the tissues, sometimes
with calcium deposits.

Variations in protraction of single doses (differences in the dose rate in terms of rad
per min) seem to have little influence on the spermatogenic effect unless the protraction
is extreme, in which case the effect of a given dose may be decreased. Such a decreased
effect probably results because cellular recovery processes are permitted to operate at
a more favorable rate with respect to the rate of production of radiation injury.

The effect of fractionation of dose on the testes is variable and depends on the size
of the total dose, the size of the dose fraction, and the length of time between fractions.
Extreme fractionation may diminish injury, the fractionation of a small dose may not
influence substantially its effect, but certain modes of fractionation of larger doses
may be more effective in damaging the spermatogenic epithelium and may more effi-
ciently damage the mechanisms responsible for restitution; that is, permanent sterility
may be caused by smaller total doses with efficient modes of fractionation than with
a single exposure. These effects of fractionation are well illustrated by data from experiments on beagles,[43,46] which show that: (1) daily (five days per week) 10-min exposures to X-rays of 0.06 or 0.12 R (150 R and 300 R, respectively, in 10 years) caused

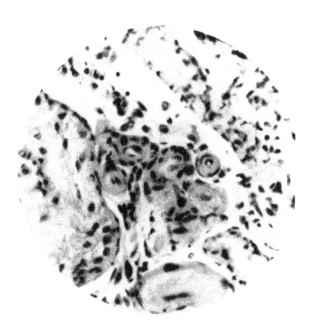

FIGURE 5A. Sections of rat testes long after permanently sterilizing radiation doses. A. Section (approximately 400×) showing marked sclerotic thickening of small blood vessels, with partial or complete occulusion of lumens. (From Casarett, G. W., *Radiat. Res. Suppl.*, 5, 246, 1964. With permission.)

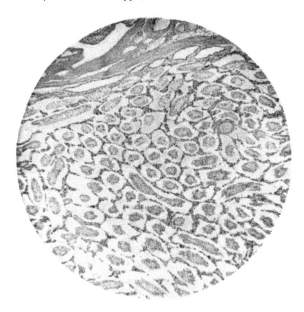

FIGURE 5B. Section (approximately 50×) showing marked atrophy and spatial condensation of tubules with fluid-filled peritibular spaces. (H. and E. stains.) (From Casarett, G. W., *Radiat. Res. Suppl.*, 5, 246, 1964. With permission.)

no reduction of sperm production or significant change in sperm quality; (2) 0.6 R per day (3 R per week) caused a reduction of sperm production and increased numbers of nonmotile, dead and abnormal spermia, with sperm counts reduced to less than 10%

of normal within a year and subsequently to zero; (3) that single doses as large as 2000 R failed to cause complete and permanent aspermia; (4) and that a total cumulated dose of about 475 R or larger administered at the rate of 3 R per day (in 10 min), 5 days per week, caused complete and permanent aspermia in 100% of the dogs.[46]

Theoretically, in tissue such as the germinal epithelium in which the stem cells (type A spermatogonia) are frequently dividing and radiosensitive, the modes of fractionation most efficient in the killing and depletion of the stem cells may be those in which the dose-time relationships are such that there is a maximum degree of mitosis-linked cell death, with a minimum of wasted radiation in respect to this efficient mechanism. Such dose-time relationships would permit quickly renewed attempts at division in radiation-injured spermatogonia, but with relatively large numbers of cells dying in preparation for or attempting division; a subsequent dose fraction would be administered when the effect of the previous dose fraction was diminishing and in time to repeat the maximal effect in the next cell generation cycle (which would tend to become more synchronized in cell generation cycle phase as a result of the earlier radiation exposure). A change in the size of the fraction or in the time interval between fractions from the most efficient dose-time relationship will theoretically decrease the efficiency of the irradiation in causing death and depletion of the stem cells. Since the population of type A spermatogonia comprises two subpopulations, differing considerably in duration of intermitotic period and in radiosensitivity, the most efficient fractionation schedule for complete and permanent sterilization of the seminiferous epithelium must be that for efficient destruction of the type A spermatogonia with the longer intermitotic periods, that is, those cells which initiate each spermatogenic cycle.

The pertinent data from human survivors of radiation accidents suggest that regeneration of spermatogenic epithelium, after marked but impermanent arrest of spermatogenesis, begins at some time between the 10th and 20th month after a single dose of radiation, and that the rate of recovery is much slower than in the small laboratory animals studied. With doses of radiation causing marked but impermanent depletion of spermatogenic epithelium, regeneration of spermatogenic epithelium may begin during the second year after radiation and possibly even later. Regeneration beginning so long after irradiation is likely to be slow and incomplete. With doses which do not permit substantial recovery of spermatogenesis, the histopathologic picture becomes one of progressive atrophy, vascular sclerosis, and replacement fibrosis.

Testes which have recovered partially or nearly completely from marked and temporary depletion of spermatogenic epithelium nevertheless show some degree of residual vascular damage and fibrosis. These changes, inherently progressive and/or added to similar changes occurring with increasing age, lead eventually to a second phase of gradual atrophy of the spermatogenic epithelium.

There is considerable delay (three weeks to two months, depending on the species) in the active regeneration of spermatogonia from those spermatogonia which evidently persist after irradiation doses that temporarily deplete the spermatogenic epithelium, but permit complete or nearly complete recovery. At low dose levels, sparing many spermatogonia, the ultimate reconstitution of the cell population appears to be primarily homeotypic, i.e., by division of persisting spermatogonia. At higher dose levels, which apparently deplete spermatogonia, but which permit eventual reconstitution of the spermatogenic epithelium after very long periods of time (many months or even years), the primary source of regenerated epithelium and even of the seemingly persisting spermatogonia is not entirely clear. Some investigators think that these spermatogonia were of a resistant type and survived, although mitosis was inhibited in them for a long time. Others have regarded these so-called persisting spermatogonia as having been derived from Sertoli cells or from undifferentiated capsular or basement membrane or interstitial cells, on the basis of observation of transitional forms. Although there is no completely satisfactory proof for any of these sources of regeneration under these conditions, the possible neoformation of new spermatogonia by transformation from more radioresistant fixed stem cells under conditions of depletion of free stem cells could help to explain the long delays in the regeneration of spermatogonia and the great difference between temporarily sterilizing doses and permanently sterilizing doses for species showing much evidence of such transitional forms, as compared with the smaller differences between such doses in species showing little evidence of such cellular transformations.

After the irradiation of the testes with a sterilizing dose, fertility may persist until there has been maturation depletion of spermatogenic cells and spermia from the genital tract to a degree sufficient to cause sterility. The duration of this initial postirradiation period of fertility depends on the duration of the spermatogenic process and the time taken for passage through the excretory ducts of the last sperm cells produced, unless massive doses affecting the fertilizing capacity of the relatively mature cells have been used.

In fixed postmitotic cells, such as spermatids and spermia, there is no opportunity to eliminate cells containing marked radiation-induced chromosomal abnormalities by the process of mitosis-linked necrosis. Consequently, conception during this early postirradiation period of fertility is associated with a relatively high probability of lethal or serious nonlethal abnormalities in the conceptus, which could become manifest in the form of an increased incidence of spontaneous abortion or in abnormalities or death of the offspring. The fertile period following the period of radiation-induced sterility, if recovery occurs, is due to spermia that were developed from cells which were spermatogonia at the time of irradiation. Conception during this period carries with it much less risk of abnormality or death of the conceptus or offspring, probably because of the death of many of the primitive cells that were rendered seriously abnormal by irradiation in their subsequent attempts to divide, and possibly in part by the recovery of some of the cells from some of their injuries by the time they become mature spermia.

Protracted or repetitive irradiation at low daily dose rates appears to be much less effective in producing abnormal, abortive, or dying embryos and offspring in experimental studies. A possible explanation for this lies in the fact that with fractionation or protraction of dose, relatively small doses are delivered to sperm populations which are continually renewed in the genitalia, so that relatively fewer spermia, with respect to the number in any one given ejaculate, are subjected to cumulative doses as large as the total accumulated dose in question. Concomitant with this, many of the spermia in each ejaculate are derived from cells which receive part of their radiation exposure as more primitive spermatogenic cells.

The so-called sterile period after irradiation may be a period of complete sterility, or a period of subfertility or fertility with reduced spermatogenesis. Since fairly large minimal numbers of normal potentially effective spermia per ejaculate are necessary for a state of fertility (high probability of fertilization), practical sterility or infertility may be associated with considerable but subnormal degrees of sperm production. When spermatogenesis is partially arrested by irradiation, aside from the reduction in the number of spermia produced, the number of potentially effective spermia is further reduced by increases in the number of spermia which are nonmotile, abnormal in various ways, or dead.

## II. THE OVARIES

In the female, as contrasted with the male, radiation destruction of the relatively

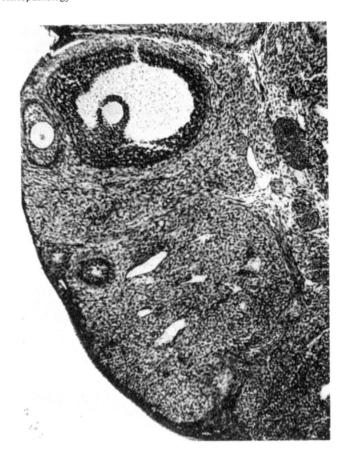

FIGURE 6.    Sections of normal rat ovaries. Approximately 200×. A.
Section showing developing follicles of various sizes.

sensitive gametogenic epithelium reduces not only gamete production, but the production of sex hormones, directly as a result of follicular destruction and indirectly in that follicular destruction reduces the precursors of the more radioresistant hormone-producing cells ordinarily derived from follicular remains after ovulation or atresia. Consequently, in the female the process of radiation sterilization of the gonads may cause the production of an artificial menopause with marked secondary effects on the more radioresistant secondary genitalia and sexual characteristics. In contrast, in the radiation destruction of spermatogenic epithelium, the separate and more independent radioresistant interstitial male sex cells are spared, and there is little or no secondary effect on secondary sexual apparatus or characteristics.

The cortical connective tissue of the ovaries contains the ovarian follicles which are of various sizes and in various stages of development and contain the ovocytes (Figure 6). Unlike the male gonad with its continuous production of spermatogonia throughout life, the production of oogonia is probably complete by the time of birth or shortly thereafter. Most of the ovarian follicles are small, primitive follicles located mainly in the peripheral cortex, and consisting of a primary oocyte surrounded by a layer of flattened granulosa cells. These give rise throughout life to all of the larger developing follicles. The primary oocyte is analogous to the primary spermatocyte. After birth, a human female starts out with a limited number of primary oocytes and ovarian follicles (perhaps one-half million) and the number is progressively reduced with the passage of time, mainly through involution or atresia of follicles (degeneration and disappear-

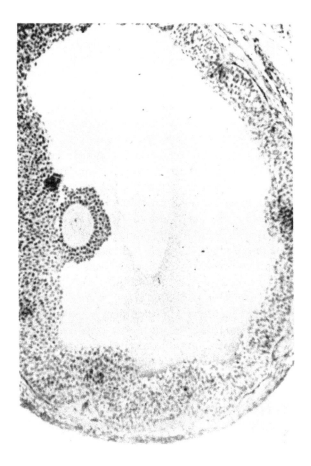

FIGURE 6B.   Section showing fully developed (Graafian) follicle virtually ready for ovulation. (H. and E. stains.)

ance), which begins in utero and is completed after the menopause. The process of ovulation once a month during the period of sexual activity accounts for the loss of only several hundred ova and follicles. Since the process of involution of follicles may start at any stage of follicular development, the normal ovary contains degenerating follicles in various sizes or stages of development.

The ova of the adult mammalian ovary are primary oocytes, homologous to primary spermatocytes, and some are in a growth and development phase. As in the case of spermatogenesis, after the primary oocyte grows, it undergoes two maturation divisions (meiosis). In the case of oogenesis, however, only one of the four potential daughter cells becomes a mature haploid ovum, while the others degenerate as abortive or rudimentary structures (polar bodies). The first of the meiotic divisions begins just before ovulation, and the second begins immediately after the expulsion of one of the secondary oocytes (first polar body) resulting fom the first division. The completion of division may be held up until after sperm penetration, or even later.

Proliferating oogonia found in intrauterine life and perhaps for a short time thereafter, originally derived from primordial germ cells, are vegetative and differentiating intermitotic cells, and are highly sensitive to the direct destructive actions of ionizing radiation. After the oogonial divisions, the oogonia become primary oocytes, which enter the prophase of meiosis before birth. Thereafter, except for those oocytes undergoing meiotic divisions immediately before ovulation, all the oocytes in follicles of any size remain in a prolonged diplotene stage, having already gone through the leptotene, zygotene, and pachytene stages. Although primary oocytes may differ in their reaction to irradiation according to the stage of meiotic prophase at exposure, in general, these cells as well as secondary oocytes are relatively radioresistant as compared with oogonia. From experimental work it would appear that the radiosensitivity of primary oocytes may decrease progressively between the leptotene and diplotene stages as meiotic prophase advances, with the trend reversing sharply at the early diplotene stage, when they become enveloped within primordial follicles. As they enter the rapid phase of growth, the sensitivity of the primary oocyte decreases again. Growing oocytes at the diplotene stage are relatively resistant to cell killing by irradiation.

Mandl[269] has reported that in rats the majority of primordial oocytes were eliminated within 18 hr after a dose of 300 rads to the ovaries, whereas slightly larger oocytes, surrounded by a single layer of cuboidal granulosa cells, were relatively insensitive in that 26% survived for 4 days after exposure to 4400 rads. The specialized connective tissue cells of the theca, the interstitial cells, and the cells of the corpora lutea behave as reverting postmitotic cells and are relatively radioresistant.

One of the most significant direct pathologic effects of radiation on the growing ovarian follicle seems to be the effect on the granulosa cells, chiefly during their period of active proliferation. During the period of active mitotic proliferation of granulosa cells, in follicles intermediate in size and development between the early follicular stage (oocytes surrounded by a single layer of granulosa cells) and the late follicular stage (Graafian follicle), the proliferating granulosa cells are vegetative intermitotic cells and relatively radiosensitive. As supporting elements of the oocytes, their damage or destruction may have profound effect on the viability of the oocytes.

In general, in growing follicles after irradiation, histopathologic damage to granulosa cells is often seen before changes in the oocyte. Pyknosis and other degenerative changes in granulosa cells become marked within the first day after moderate radiation doses (e.g., 750 rads) to the rat ovary (Figures 7A and 7B). By the 25th day after irradiation, there is marked reduction in the number of developing follicles (Figure 7C) and considerable increase in vacuolization of cells in the corpora lutea secondary to the follicular effect (Figures 7C and 7D).

With doses small enough to spare many granulosa cells and their ability to resume proliferation, the granulosa cell layer may recover rapidly. With larger doses, causing greater damage to granulosa cells and preventing such rapid regeneration, the oocyte degenerates, and the follicle undergoes further changes, similar at least in some respects to atresia, and becomes atrophic.

In the case of temporary radiation-induced sterility of the female, the initial fertile period after irradiation and before the sterility period is due to the persistence of follicles in the late, relatively radioresistant stages of development at the time of irradiation, when granulosa cell proliferation has subsided. The period of temporary sterility which follows this initial fertile period is the result of radiation destruction of the relatively radiosensitive follicles of intermediate size and development, in which there is intensive granulosa cell proliferation. The fertile period after recovery from the sterile period is the result of the development of mature follicles from relatively radioresistant primitive follicles, that were small, with little or no granulosa cell proliferation, at the time of irradiation. Since there are no stem cells analogous to the type A spermatogonia of the male, presumably the radiation destruction of follicles may result in a permanent premature decline in the number of available or potential follicles. After recovery from radiation effects it is possible also that there may be some residual effect in the form of an increased rate of atresia of the remaining follicles.

Experimental work to date on mice following irradiation at different dose rates indicates that lower dose rates permit greater survival of oocytes and greater reproductive

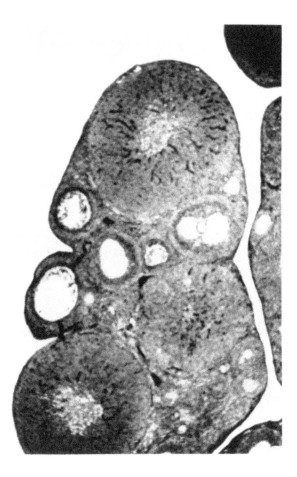

FIGURE 7. Sections of rat ovaries after 750R of X-rays. A. Section (approximately 100×) one day after irradiation, showing marked degeneration or necrosis of granulosa cells in the developing follicles, apparent loss of oocytes from some of the follicles, and vacuolation of cells in the corpora lutea.

capacity. Experimental work on rats has suggested that whole-body irradiation may cause greater destruction of follicles than irradiation of the ovaries alone with similar doses.

An experimental study of the total population of oocytes in adult rats after irradiation[267] has shown that exposure to doses of 31, 78, 315, and 630 R was followed many months later (mean 288 days) by a reduction in the number of oocytes to 83, 51, 4, and 1%, respectively, of that of the control population.

After radiation doses causing permanent and complete sterility, the ovaries reveal complete or nearly complete absence of primordial follicles, continued decrease of residual remains of follicles undergoing atrophy, and degeneration and decrease of the corpora lutea and interstitial gland cells, together with progressive vascular sclerosis and replacement fibrosis.

Following substantial doses of radiation which do not cause permanent sterility, there is a residual increase in genic or chromosomal abnormalities in oocytes. In addition to the possibility of genic abnormalities in the offspring, some of these abnormalities may become manifest in the form of an increased incidence of abortion. Van Wagenen and Gardner[276] have shown that a single X-ray dose of 600 rads to the ovaries

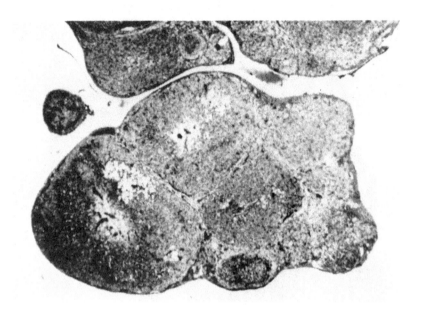

FIGURE 7C.    Section (approximately 100×) 25 days after irradiation, showing virtual absence of normal developing follicles and the persistence of vacuolation of cells of corpora lutea.

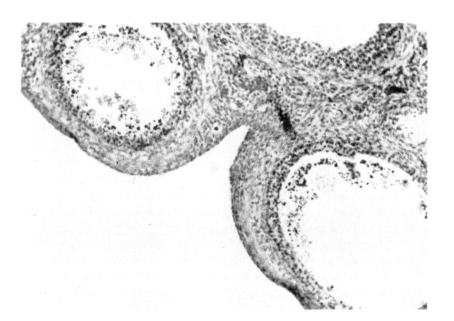

FIGURE 7B.    Section (approx. 200×) one day after irradiation, showing cellular debris from necrotic granulosa cells in developing follicles and the degnerate remains of an oocyte in one of the follicles (lower left).

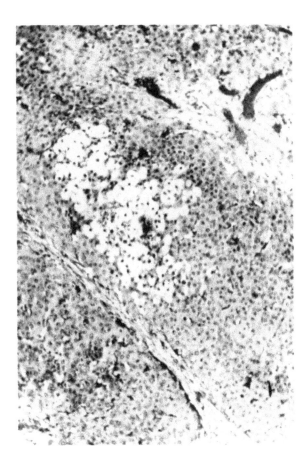

FIGURE 7D.   Section (approximagely 200×) 25 days after irradiation, showing vacuolization of cells of corpora lutea. (H.
and E. stains.)

of monkeys did not cause appreciable irregularity of the menstrual cycle for periods
up to 10 years, that pregnancy occurred when the irradiated monkeys were mated although the incidence of conception was reduced, and that 20 of 21 pregnancies termi-
nated in abortion, most frequently between the 39th and 49th day after conception.

Chapter 6

# BONE AND CARTILAGE

## I. MATURE BONE AND CARTILAGE

### A. Histology

Bone is the most highly differentiated and specialized of the supporting or connective tissues. It is a hard rigid tissue consisting of a relatively great volume of calcified collagenous intercellular matrix, with inorganic salts in the ground substance, and relatively few cells. Most bones of the body contain both compact external (cortical) bone (Figure 1A) and internal cancellous (spongy) bone (Figure 1B) with marrow in its spaces. Both types of bone are composed of the same histologic elements in different arrangements.

Bones are covered externally by the periosteum, a specialized connective tissue sheath with a dense, vascular, fibrous (mostly collagenous) outer layer and a less dense, more elastic, and cellular inner layer. The inner layer is most distinct during developmental periods or, in the adults, when stimulated (e.g., by fracture), when osteoblasts (bone forming cells) are prominent in this layer. Vessels and nerves pass through the periosteum to the bone. The marrow spaces within bones are surrounded by endosteum, a delicate connective tissue layer similar to the periosteum in its bone forming and dissolving capabilities. The endosteum covers the surface of spongy bone, lines the internal surfaces of compact bone, and extends into the canal system of compact bone. It also has hematopoietic potential.

Bone develops by ossification of connective tissue (intramembraneous ossification), by osseous transformation or replacement of cartilage (intracartilagenous or endochondral ossification), or by a combination of these two processes. Bone tissue is formed by the process of apposition of new bone upon connective tissue, cartilage, or bone. Each of the three types of bone cells (osteoblast, osteocyte, and osteoclast) can undergo transformation to the other types, and each can be formed by transformation from, and can transform to, mesenchymal cells, fibroblasts, and reticular cells. These three types of bone cells divide rarely under normal conditions and are relatively resistant to the direct destructive actions of radiation. The bone-forming cells (osteoblasts) are found on the surface of developing and growing bone and may be involved in the synthesis of the proteins of the bone matrix. The bone cells proper (osteocytes) are formed from osteoblasts that have become surrounded by bone matrix. During the early stages of development of bone, fine cytoplasmic processes of the osteocytes extend through canaliculi (fine capillary tubes) radiating from osteocyte spaces (lacunae) to interconnect with cytoplasmic processes from other osteocytes in other lacunae. Some open into periosteal and endosteal surfaces, and others open into haversian canals. However, in the mature bone of mammals, these cytoplasmic processes appear to have withdrawn markedly, and it is not known how far they extend into the canaliculi. The cells associated with resorption of bone, the osteoclasts, are multinucleated giant cells which are derived from stromal cells of marrow and possibly can be formed by fusion of osteoblasts.

The hard matrix or calcified interstitial substance of bone, the greater part of bone, is composed of an organic framework component, including osteocollagenous fibers cemented by a special mucoalbuminoid primary ground substance, and an inorganic component of bone salt (chiefly submicroscopic crystals of calcium phosphate with the structure of an apatite mineral) deposited in this cement substance.

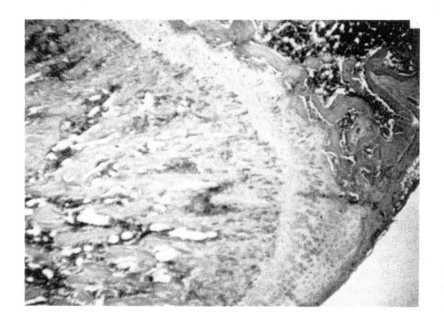

FIGURE 1B. Section (approximately 100×) of distal rat femur (H. and E. stains), showing the epiphysial spongy bone and marrow (bottom) separated from the metaphysial spongy bone (top) by the horizontal cartilage plate (physis) of the zone of endochondral bone growth.

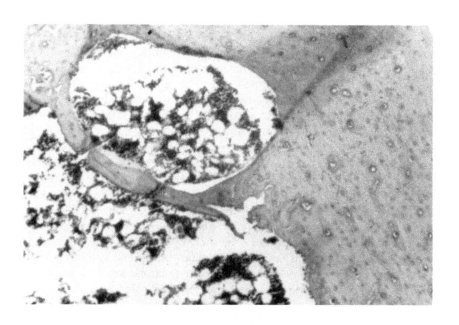

FIGURE 1. Sections of normal bone. A. Section (approximately 200×) of rat femoral cortical bone (H. & E. stains) showing osteocytes in their lacunae.

97

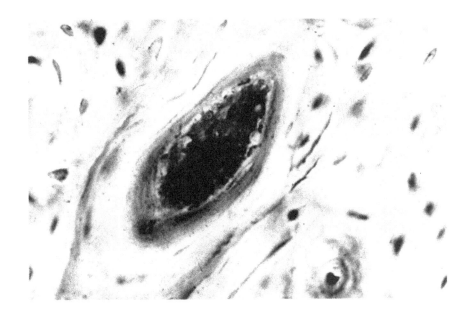

FIGURE 1D. Section of normal rabbit tibial cortex (approximately 1000×; H. and E. stains) showing a forming osteon (center) and surrounding lamellae with osteocytes in lacunae. (C and D from King, M. and Casarett, G. W., unpublished).

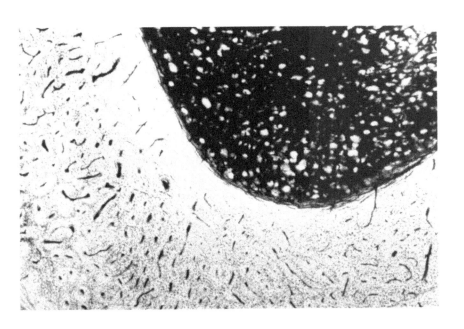

FIGURE 1C. Ultraviolet photomicrograph of a section of normal cortex of rabbit tibia (approximately 100×) showing haversian systems (osteons) and canals of Volkmann as well as the very small dots indicating osteocytic lacunae.

In bone growth, bone matrix is deposited in layers (lamellae) 3 to 7 $\mu$m thick and arranged in flat or curved (concentric) parallel series. Lamellae are arranged in sets (haversian systems, periosteal and endosteal lamellae, interstitial lamellae) which are separated from one another by thin refractile cement membranes (Figure 1C). Bone undergoes internal remodeling throughout life.

The internal structure of compact bone differs from that of spongy bone in the development of haversian systems (osteons) as the structural units of compact bone (Figure 1D). The osteons are oriented chiefly to the long axis of the bone. The axis of an haversian system is the haversian canal (generally from 22 to 110 $\mu$m in diameter), which contains within its loose connective tissue one or more blood vessels (mostly capillaries and postcapillary venules, occasionally an arteriole), lymphatics, and nerves. Each haversian canal is surrounded by from 4 to 20 concentrically arranged lamellae. Each osteon contains large numbers of osteocytes in their individual lacunae, and the extravascular canaliculi radiating from the canal and interconnecting with the lacunae and other canaliculi of the osteon. Tissue fluids diffuse between the vessels in the canal and the osteocytic and lamellar surfaces through these canaliculi. Haversian canals often open into the marrow cavity.

The irregular regions between osteons are filled by interstitial (ground) lamellae, mostly remnants of osteons partly destroyed during internal remodeling. The haversian systems are bounded near the external and internal surfaces of compact bone by the basic outer and inner circumferential lamellae. The canals of Volkmann, which contain the blood vessels (usually larger than those of the haversian system) communicating with those in the haversian canals, pass through these lamellae and open at the external and internal (marrow cavity) surfaces of the bone. The blood vessels of the periosteum that connect with those in the haversian canals do so via the canals of Volkmann.

In general, the arterial supply to bones is provided by arterioles which enter the bone from the periosteum. These and their capillary branches pass through the Volkmann and haversian canals and reach the marrow. Some of the venules retrace the arterial course. These arterioles and venules are mostly thin-walled, like capillaries in structure. In addition, in long bones one or more large arteries enter the bones at about midshaft, pass obliquely to the marrow in a prominent canal and give rise to proximal and distal branches. Although corresponding veins retrace this arterial course, most of the blood of the spongy bone and marrow is returned through numerous veins that leave the bone at its extremities. Even though bone contains many small blood vessels, there are no capillary networks within the bone matrix. In compact bone, the blood vessels are limited to the external and internal surfaces and the conducting canals within the bone, and in spongy bone to the marrow spaces between bone structures. The fluid in the canaliculi provides for diffusion of gases, nutrients, and catabolic wastes between osteocytes in their lacunae and lamellar surfaces and the vessels in the canals, but the dense bone matrix does not permit the diffusion of these substances through it. The vasculature in bone is a relatively fixed system compared to that in most soft tissue and does not permit as much flexibility in the development of collateral circulation.

Bone tissue (bone cells and matrix) does not replace itself directly nor repair local injuries or gross fractures by itself, but repair is achieved through the actions of associated tissues. Upon fracture of a bone there is hemorrhage from torn vessels, and the organization of the clotted blood by granulation tissue (proliferating fibroblasts and budding capillaries) forms a procallous. This substance consolidates, and cartilage develops within it to form the temporary or fibrocartilagenous callous, which fills in the gap and unites the broken ends of the bone. The newly formed bone that will eventually unite the fractured ends begins to form at a distance from the fracture, starting with the appearance of osteoblasts in the deep layer of the periosteum and in the en-

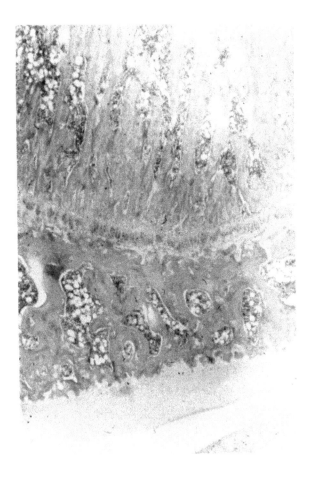

FIGURE 2. Sections showing normal mature rat cartilage. A. Femoral-tibial joint cartilage (bottom). Approximately 50×.

dosteum. Spongy bone is formed, gradually replaces the fibrocartilagenous callous with a bony callous, achieves bony union, and reorganizes into compact bone.

Cartilage is a specialized type of dense fibrous connective tissue consisting of cells and matrix (fibers and ground substance) that forms most of the temporary skeleton of the fetus, provides a base or template for the development of most bones, and persists in adults as parts of joints (Figure 2A), respiratory passages (Figure 2B), and the ears. Like bone, the volume of intercellular matrix of cartilage is much greater than the total volume of the cartilage cells (chondrocytes). Unlike bone, cartilage contains no intrinsic blood vessels, lymphatics, or nerves, although blood vessels sometimes pass through cartilage on their way to other tissues. As there are no canaliculi in the matrix, nutrients, oxygen, and cell wastes must diffuse through the matrix between perichondrial blood vessels and chondrocytes.

Except for the noncovered surfaces of joint cartilage, cartilage is encased by dense collagenous connective tissue (perichondrium). The perichondrial tissue nearest the cartilage is more cellular, with relatively young, flattened cells intermediate in form between cartilage cells and fibroblasts. The cartilage cells under the free surface of the joint are also flattened, but the chondrocytes deeper in the cartilage tend to be spherical in shape, although sometimes distorted by pressure. In the adult the chondrocytes rarely have cytoplasmic extensions like those of osteocytes.

During its development the cartilage grows interstitially, i.e., by mitotic production

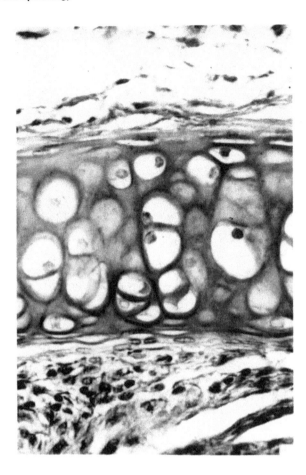

FIGURE 2B.  Tracheal cartilage bounded by perichondrial
connective tissue. Approximately 800×. (H. and E. stains.)

of groups of chondrocytes in the matrix and separation of the cells by the new matrix
formed by them, and by appositional growth, i.e., by the transformation of perichondrial fibroblasts into cartilage cells which deposit a matrix about themselves. In mature
cartilage, after growth has ceased, the adult chondrocytes rarely divide and may be
regarded as reverting postmitotic cells. They are relatively resistant to the direct destructive actions of radiation. Injuries or losses of mature cartilage are not repaired
by the cartilage itself, but the defect is filled by connective tissue newly formed from
the perichondrium or nearby fascia. Fibroblasts of this connective or granulation tissue
become transformed to chondrocytes which deposit new cartilage matrix about themselves. The fibrillar interstitial material of the scar tissue becomes homogenous and
gives rise to new interstitial substance. A fracture of mature cartilage sometimes becomes united by permanent fibrous tissue, and sometimes some of its fibrous tissue is
replaced by bone rather than cartilage.

## B. Radiation Histopathology

Early after irradiation, substantial degrees of radiation damage in mature bone and
cartilage are relatively subtle and difficult to detect, as compared with many kinds of
soft tissues sustaining equivalent damage. This is a result of the relative paucity of
cells, the abundance of matrix, the radioresistance of the matrix and the mature cells,
and the normally slow turnover or metabolism of the greater part of the matrix, i.e.,

the part more remote from blood vessels and active cells. Gross changes, e.g., roentgenographic changes, in the matrix of these tissues after irradiation are relatively slow to develop for some of these reasons, i.e., because of the maintenance of macroscopic or structural integrity of the mineralized matrix for long periods of time in regions of low metabolic rate or turnover.

The nonproliferating bone and cartilage cells are relatively resistant to the direct cytocidal actions of radiation. The bulk of evidence indicates that the principal factor in radiation damage to mature bone or cartilage is the damage to the fine vasculature supplying these structures, with the degeneration and loss of dependent cells being secondary to interference with blood supply, and with changes in the matrix being secondary to either or both of these changes. In the case of mature bone, the damage to the intraosseous vasculature, with occlusion of the fine vasculature and canals or canaliculi, secondary loss of osteocytes, and the damage to the periosteal vasculature and to osteoblasts, are of prime importance in the pathogenesis of radiation- nduced damage. In the case of mature cartilage also, which does not contain the fine vasculature within it and which is regenerated by fibroblasts from the surrounding perichondrium or connective tissue, the radiation damage to the surrounding fine vasculature and connective tissue (perichondritis) is of prime importance in the development of radiation damage in the cartilage.

Minor damage to the vasculature or to the cell population in mature bone or cartilage may cause little or no visible change in the matrix at early times after irradiation. Rapid recovery from such damage may prevent even the temporary appearance of secondary effects in regions of the matrix which have a low metabolic rate. Large degrees of vascular damage and secondary degeneration and disappearance of many of the bone or cartilage cells are eventually reflected in gradual changes in the matrix. However for a considerable period of time after irradiation, the difference between viable and nonviable bone or cartilage, aside from the vascular and cellular changes, may consist only of slight differences in staining characteristics and mineralization of the matrix. In time, with persistence or progression of occlusion of the fine vasculature and secondary degeneration and loss of parenchymal cells, the bone matrix shows gradually increasing resorption of osteons (Figure 3), disorganization of structure, porosis, and fibrosis. Analogous effects occur in cartilage in so-called radiation chondritis (Figure 4).

Whether or when such devitalization of bone or cartilage results in frank necrosis, i.e., structural disintegration, depends upon the degree of initial vascular damage and the rate of progression of occlusion of the fine vasculature and secondary loss of parenchymal cells, and also upon the occurrence of complicating factors such as trauma or infection. With advanced progression of obliterative vascular lesions and loss of cells, aseptic necrosis of the bone or cartilage may occur. Or, as a result of the increased susceptibility of such damaged tissues to infection, complicating infection may cause septic necrosis, with disintegration of the structures in the areas affected. Sequestration in such radionecrotic areas is slower than in areas of necrosis caused by only trauma or infection. Since radiation damage retards the repair of bone or cartilage after damage from trauma or infection, regeneration of irradiated necrotic areas may fail to occur or may be very slow and far from complete.

As is the case with other tissues in which the parenchymal cells are more radioresistant than the fine vasculature, aseptic radionecrosis of bone or cartilage may be caused early by large doses that cause marked damage to the vasculature and early marked loss of osteocytes or chondrocytes, or later by small doses as a result of the more slowly progressive reduction of blood supply and loss of parenchymal cells. The intraosseous vasculature is a relatively fixed system with respect to flexibility and the

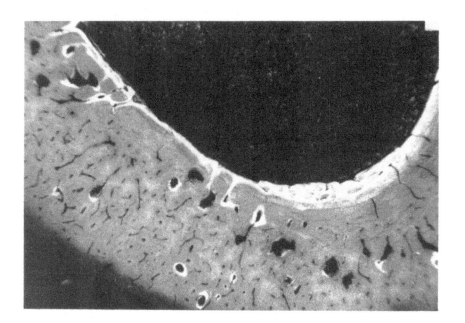

FIGURE 3B.    Section three months after 1756 rads, showing excessive resorption of osteons and porosity of bone.

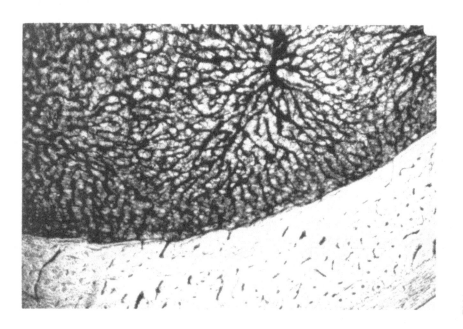

FIGURE 3.    Ultraviolet photomicrographs of rabbit tibial cortex. Approximately 100×. A. Normal cortical bone for comparison.

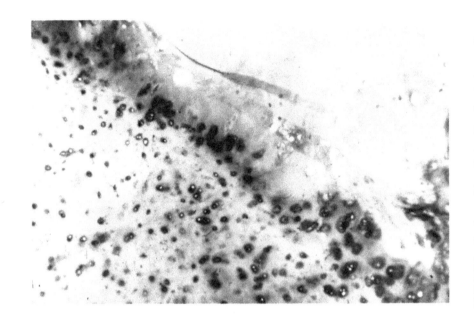

FIGURE 4. Sections of heavily irradiated articular cartilage. A. Partial necrosis secondary to radiation damage of vascular supply (approximately 400×).

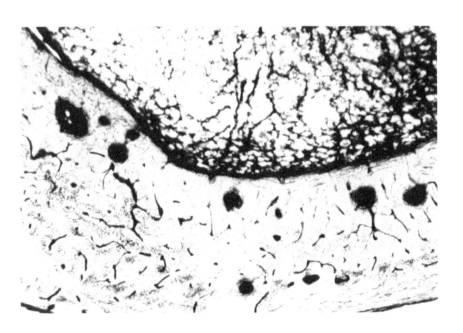

FIGURE 3C. Section 6 months after 1756 rads, showing excessive resorption of osteons and disorganization of bone remodeling. (From King, M. and Casarett, G. W., unpublished).

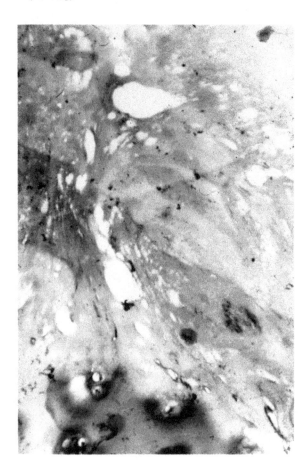

FIGURE 4B.   Higher magnification (approximately 800×) of part of the section in A, showing necrosis of chondrocytes in lacunae (bottom) adjacent to the frankly necrotic area. (H. and E. stains.)

development of collateral circulation, as compared with the fine vasculature within most soft tissues, so that recovery of intraosseous circulation after radiation damage tends to be slow and far from complete.

## II. ENDOCHONDRAL BONE GROWTH

### A. Histology

The process of endochondral bone growth is radiosensitive because of the radiosensitivity of growing cartilage and bone marrow. Endochondral bone growth, i.e., bone growth in the wake of growth of cartilage is described here as exemplified in the longitudinal growth of the rat femur. The normal disc of hyaline cartilage (physis) in the center of endochondral bone growth, situated horizontally between the bony plate of the epiphysis and the cancellous bone of the metaphysis, may be described in terms of five zones, proceeding from the bony plate of the epiphysis to the metaphysis (Figure 5A):

**Zone 1** — This zone, adjacent to the bony plate of the epiphysis, contains reserve, resting chondroblasts which behave as reverting postmitotic cells in that they divide infrequently under normal conditions, but can proliferate under appropriate stimulus. These cells are relatively resistant to the direct cytocidal actions of radiation.

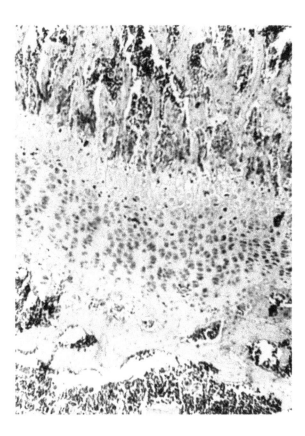

FIGURE 5. Sections of distal femurs of rats in the zone of endochondral longitudinal bone growth after 750R of X-rays. A. Normal section for comparison, showing columns of cartilage cells (center) between the metaphysial spongiosa (above) and the epiphysial spongiosa below.

**Zone 2** — This is the zone of proliferation of chondroblasts in longitudinal columns. In the longitudinally growing bone, the chondroblasts of this zone behave as vegetative intermitotic cells, dividing frequently to produce daughter cells, some of which remain as vegetative intermitotic cells, and some of which grow and differentiate in the subsequent zones of the columns. These vegetative intermitotic chondroblasts are relatively radiosensitive.

**Zone 3** — In this zone the differentiating chondroblasts increase in size, but do not undergo further division. They behave under normal conditions as reverting or fixed postmitotic cells and are relatively radioresistant.

**Zone 4** — In this zone the cartilage cells and their lacunae are fully developed, and there is mineralization of the hyaline cartilage matrix, especially that between the columns of cartilage cells. These cartilage cells are also relatively radioresistant.

**Zone 5** — This is the zone in which calcified primary cartilagenous trabeculae (primary spongiosa) are formed by invasion of the columns of cartilage cells by the cells and vasculature of the primary metaphysial marrow. Osteoblasts become applied to the surface of the primary cartilagenous trabeculae and osteoid material is formed on these trabeculae. With subsequent mineralization of the osteoid material and differentiation of entrapped cells in lacunae to osteocytes, true bone is formed, as may be seen in the osseous trabeculae of the secondary spongiosa in the metaphysis closer to the diaphasis (shaft). Osteoclasts applied to the trabeculae are associated with resorption of excess bone in the metaphysis, so that under normal conditions trabecular bone

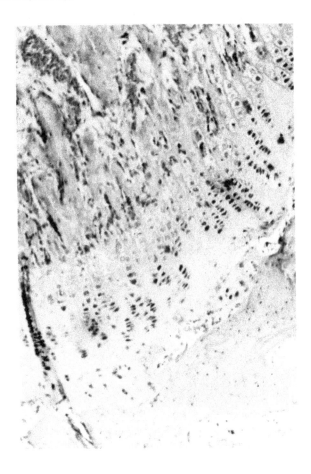

FIGURE 5B.   Section three days after irradiation, showing
decrease in number of chondroblasts in zone of proliferation
and marrow hypoplasia.

does not invade the diaphysial marrow in the process of longitudinal bone growth. The newly formed bone in the peripheral regions of the zone of endochondral ossification is added to the length of the shaft of the long bone. The osteoblasts, osteocytes, and osteoclasts are generally relatively radioresistant, since these cells are reverting postmitotic cells. The fine vasculature of the primary metaphasial marrow is moderately radiosensitive, and the proliferating cells of the marrow are relatively radiosensitive.

In the eventual cessation of bone growth at epiphysial centers, the processes of proliferation of cartilage cells and vascular invasion of the cartilage cease gradually, bone is deposited at the metaphysial margin of the cartilage disc, and there may be varying degrees of replacement of the cartilage disc by bone, tending to make the cancellous bone of the epiphysial and metaphysial cavities more continuous.

## B. Radiation Histopathology

Rubin et al.[304] have experimentally produced in the growing long bones of rats a variety of bone dysplasias by irradiation of the whole bone, the epiphysis only, the metaphysis only, or the diaphysis only, with a single intensive dose of 2400 R, a dose that is capable of causing complete cessation of chondrogenesis and osteogenesis. After irradiation of the whole bone with this dose, there was initially complete cessation of

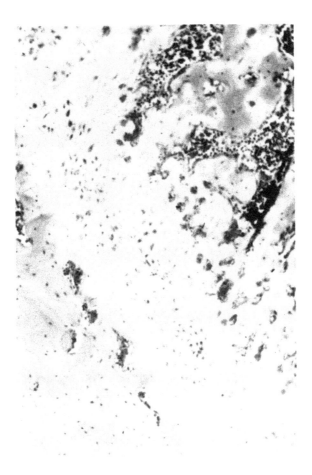

FIGURE 5C. Section 25 days after irradiation, showing marked decrease in number of cartilage cells and disorganization of the cellular columns in the cartilage plate, with thickening of the primary cartilaginous trabeculae in the metaphysis and decreased and variable deposition of osteoid material on these trabeculae. The bone marrow in the metaphysis shows considerable regeneration. (H. and E. stains; magnification approximately 200×.)

bone growth within a few days. The shaft became extremely delicate in appearance, fractured readily and resembled severe osteogenesis imperfecta on roentgenograms. With the arrest and failure of endochondral bone formation and of intramembranous appositional osteogenic processes in the diaphysis, the bones retained their narrow shape, giving the appearance of a lack of cylindrization. After irradiation of the epiphysis, including the growing cartilage plate (physis), a marked reduction in longitudinal bone growth occurred, with slight-to-marked reduction in bone width. The ultimate effect was that of dwarfing, but with normal cylindrization and with either a complete lack of funnelization or a definite flaring in the metaphysial region. After irradiation of the metaphysis, there was little stunting of longitudinal bone growth, little or no funnelization, but definite bowing. After diaphysial irradiation there was marked narrowing of the irradiated diaphysis, with normal cortical thickness, but narrowing and fibrosis of the marrow cavity and normal growth of the ends of the bone, with little or no stunting of longitudinal growth. The condition in the irradiated diaphysis may be explained by the fact that appositional intramembranous osteogenesis is more radioresistant than marrow and osteoclastic processes. The narrowed diaphysis was also the site of transverse fractures in the animals.

From experimental observations such as these and others, it is clear that the special distribution of absorbed radiation energy within bones, together with the relative radiosensitivity of osteogenic elements at the sites of energy absorption, determines the specific growth processes and sites more affected and therefore the eventual outcome as far as effects on bone growth (longitudinal by endochondral processes, or transverse by intramembranous appositional processes), bone modeling, or shape are concerned.

In general, the severity of the effect varies directly with the dose, and fractionation or protraction of the dose has been found to lessen the degree of effect. In regard to the importance of the relative radiosensitivity of osteogenic elements or processes in determining the ultimate outcome of radiation effect in growing bone, it should be emphasized that the damage to the moderately sensitive fine vasculature of the marrow, cartilage, or bone and their capability for recovery play a large role in determining the degree of recovery of bone growth processes after irradiation. Since the nondividing reserve chondroblasts of the growing physial cartilage plate are relatively radioresistant, they can initiate the regeneration of a growing cartilage plate in the event of survival or regeneration of adequate vasculature, even after severe damage to the proliferating and growing chondroblasts and devitalization of other parts of the plate. This may be associated with splitting off of the devitalized portion of the plate adjacent to the metaphysis, and displacement of this separated portion of the plate toward the diaphysis as longitudinal bone growth is resumed and progresses.

The severity and time of appearance of, and time and degree of recovery from, the histopathologic effects of irradiation in the zones of endochondral bone growth are dependent upon both dose and age at the time of irradiation, and so is the degree of stunting of bone length. Some of the factors responsible for this dependence are the greater radiosensitivity of the more rapidly proliferating chondroblasts associated with phases of rapid skeletal growth, and the greater potential for stunting of bone length in bones that are far from obtaining their full length at time of irradiation.

As a result of these differences in the radiosensitivity of the growing cartilage at different ages, the minimal dose for the production of observable histopathologic changes in the growing cartilage and the minimal stunting dose (MSD) generally tend to vary directly with age. In other words, for a given dose the degree of acute cartilage damage and of growth stunting generally varies inversely with age at irradiation, at least after organization of the growth zone has occurred. According to Hinkel,[293] the MSD for grossly appreciable stunting of bone length in long bones of rats 30 days of age is 600 R (about 10% stunting in the 1st month after irradiation) and the MSD in rats more than 4 or 5 months old is 1600 to 2000 R. The minimal dose for the production of observable histopathological changes in cartilage is in most cases about 20% below the MSD.

The high MSD in older, more slowly growing, bones causes a greater extent and degree of irreversible damage in the marrow and fine vasculature than does the lower MSD in younger, more rapidly growing bones. The rising radioresistance of the growing cartilage with increasing age is associated with a lesser degree of change in radiosensitivity of the marrow and fine vasculature with age. Consequently, the MSD for the slowly growing bones may result in lesser degrees of recovery of the growing cartilage and the bone-growth process than the lower MSD for rapidly growing bones, by virtue of the relatively greater damage to the fine vasculature in the former instance.

After irradiation with the MSD, young or rapidly growing bones reveal histopathologic changes in the growing cartilage within a day or two, whereas in older animals receiving the MSD, comparable changes may not become apparent for a week or so, and the development of the damage is much slower.

For a given age, the degree of radiation effect on bone growth varies directly with the size of the dose up to a point of maximal effect, beyond which increasing dose causes no greater change in bone growth. The dose of maximal effect causes marked irreversible damage in the marrow and its fine vasculature and consequently adversely affects the recovery and growth of the cartilage in the zone of endochrondral ossification, even if there is survival of reserve chondroblasts capable of regenerating a new cartilage plate. The dose of maximal effect also varies with age, since it is a function of the combined factors of the radiosensitivities and recovery capabilities of all the elements involved in the bone-growth process.

In summary, irradiation of growing bone can cause stunting of bone growth by damaging the proliferating cartilage cells in the growing cartilage of zones of endochondral ossification and thereby causing temporary retardation or cessation of cartilage growth. After a variable interval of retardation or cessation of growth, there may be regeneration of cartilage cells and resumption of growth at a normal or retarded rate, with eventual cessation of growth at the normal time or prematurely, depending upon the interrelated factors of dose and age and upon the degree and extent of the irreversible damage to the fine vasculature and marrow. Hinkel[294,295] has demonstrated in rats a very close correlation between blood vessel recovery or regeneration and the return of bone-growth processes. When the vessels appear normal, the marrow and osteoblasts also appear normal, and chondroclastic and osteoclastic processes, new bone formation, and growth in length, all progress physiologically. The return to normal histology is much more prompt in the portions of the cartilage plate closest to the periosteal blood vessels. After doses large enough to destroy vessels and marrow cells and to prevent recovery of these elements, chondroclastic processes, bone resorption, columnar arrangement of cartilage cells in the cartilage plate, and true osteoblastic bone formation are absent or markedly deficient.

The early histopathologic effects of radiation on the growing cartilage in the zone of endochondral bone formation are evident within a few days or a week, depending upon the dose regimen. These early changes (Figure 5B) are most prominent in the zone of proliferating chondroblasts (zone 2) and include reduction of mitotic activity, degeneration and necrosis and reduction in the number of chondroblasts, enlargement of lacunae, relatively increased intercolumnar matrix, the beginning of spatial irregularity and distortion of the cell columns, and the beginning of excessive accumulation of osteoid or osseous material replacing the primary cartilagenous trabeculae or being deposited on the metaphysial trabeculae in relation to the retardation or cessation of growth-induced displacement of the trabeculae toward the diaphysis. The bone marrow reveals marked damage or hypoplasia at this time, and the associated fine vasculature is also damaged. Osteoblastic and osteoclastic processes are less affected. Subsequently these early changes become more or less manifest in degenerative changes in other parts of the cartilage plate or in metaphysial structures, depending on the dose and the rapidity and degree of recovery from acute damage. In 3 to 4 weeks after 750 R the damage of the cartilage plate has become more advanced, but the marrow cellularity and vasculature has recovered (Figures 5C).

Radiation doses of moderate size (for example 600 to 1200 rads) cause submaximal damage to the cartilage plate that varies in degree with the size of the dose. Such doses permit sufficiently rapid recovery of the chondroblasts and vasculature and of bone growth to limit the progression and accumulation of secondary changes in the cartilage plate and metaphysial bone. However some degree of residual damage, varying directly with the dose, may remain in the form of subnormal numbers of cartilage cells, a relative increase in amounts of cartilagenous matrix, irregularities in orientation of cartilage cell columns, marrow hypoplasia, and relative hypovascularity or vascular sclerosis. Once resumed, the bone-growth process may continue at a normal rate or

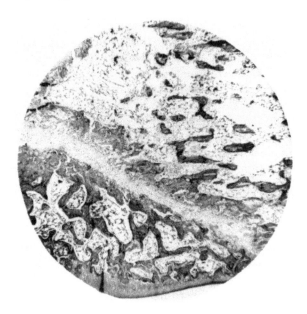

FIGURE 6.    Sections of distal femurs of rats in the zone of
endochondral longitudinal bone growth after large radiation
doses causing permanent cessation of bone growth. A. Section
(approximately 50×) about 1 month after irradiation, showing
hypoplastic marrow, cessation of production of primary cartilagenous trabeculae, conversion of existing trabeculae to osteoid or bone, and marked resorption of secondary metaphysial spongiosa.

perhaps at a somewhat reduced rate, depending upon dose size, but the temporary
interruption in bone growth results in a stunted bone, as there is no compensation for
the interruption, and the eventual cessation of bone growth occurs at the normal time,
if not prematurely.

Larger doses of radiation (for example 1800 to 3000 rads or more) cause maximal
or near maximal damage of the zone of chondroblastic proliferation (zone 2), and the
damage to the fine vasculature and bone marrow and other cellular elements of the
region is also much greater than that seen after small doses. The primitive reserve
chondroblasts in zone 1, although many may survive and show little degenerative
change, are more delayed in attempting to proliferate and replace lost chondroblasts,
partly because of the circulatory impairment. Even after the large doses that do not
permit recovery of bone growth, these reserve chondroblasts may make such attempts,
but they are abortive in that the small collections of proliferating chondroblasts produced usually fail to attain the normal columnar orientation and are surrounded by
dense devitalized cartilage that is not being invaded by vasculature.

Recovery of the fine vasculature is slow and usually far from complete after large
doses. As a result of the long delay or failure of recovery of bone growth and the
consequent cessation of displacement of primary cartilagenous trabeculae and metaphysial spongiosa, the cartilagenous matrix of the plate becomes dense and more brittle; the plate becomes flattened and narrowed; there are progressive increases in the
amounts of osteoid, osseous or bone-like material deposited on and displacing primary
cartilagenous trabeculae and on the metaphysial spongiosa; the connections between
the primary trabeculae and the cartilage plate become dissolved; and a horizontal osseous or bone-like barrier is formed along the flattened metaphysial margin of the
cartilage plate (Figure 6). This barrier is similar to that formed in the process of normal

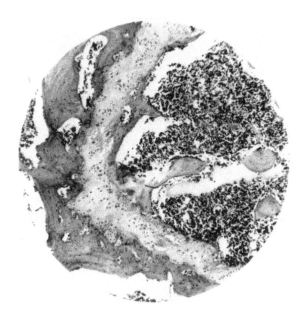

FIGURE 6B. Section (approximately 100×) about 5 months after irradiation, showing persistent marked reduction in numbers of cartilage cells in the cartilage plate, formation of an osteoid or osseous margin between the plate and the metaphysial bone marrow (which has recovered), and virtually complete absorption of metaphysial spongiosa.

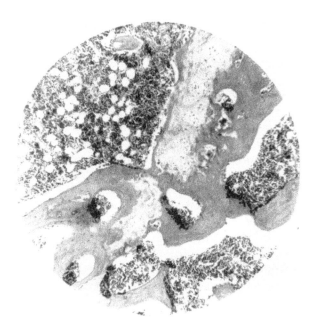

FIGURE 6C. Section (approximately 100×) more than a year after irradiation showing premature epiphysial closure with conversion of parts of the cartilage plate to bone and sealing of the plate from the metaphysis by bone.

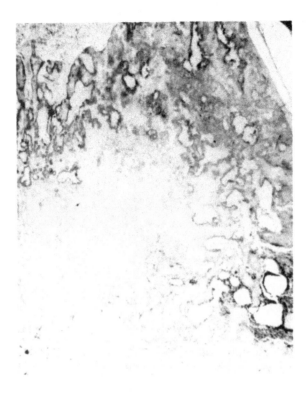

FIGURE 6D.    Overgrowth of the cartilage plate into the metaphysis with its hypoplastic, hypovascular marrow. (H. and
E. stains.) (A—D from Casarett, G. W., *Radiat. Res. Suppl.*,
5, 246, 1964. With permission.)

spontaneous cessation of bone growth. There is gradual replacement of the cartilagenous plate by bone.

The osteoblasts are much more resistant to radiation destruction than the proliferating chondroblasts, and consequently osteoid deposition and osteogenesis may continue after cartilage growth has ceased. When the radiation dose is large enough to
cause a marked deficiency or absence of osteoblasts, osteoid deposition and true osteogenesis do not occur. However, under such conditions, resistant cartilage cells in the
cartilage plate or cartilagenous trabeculae may become transformed into functioning
osteoblasts, and hyalin cartilage appears to be directly converted into bone. But most
of this material is nearly acellular and avascular and has been considered to be pseu-
dobone. Such material is dense and brittle.

The effectiveness of the chondroclastic and osteoclastic processes after irradiation
depends upon the degree of recovery of the vasculature and the marrow. These processes are deficient when the marrow cells and vessels are severely damaged. As a result
of this, foci of cartilage may persist as such far from the growth zone and become
embodied in the newly formed bone, where they may be found months later. There
may be imbalances in bone and cartilage formation and in chondroclastic and osteoclastic processes as a result of varying degrees of effects on osteoblasts, chondroblasts,
and the vasculature that may persist for months and result in irregular patterns of
changes of the kinds described. The irregular decreases in size and number of blood
vessels as a result of radiation damage cause not only irregular hypoxia, but also variable reduction in the vascular erosive function which is reflected by the migration or
overgrowth, after bone growth resumption, of unresorbed and nonossified cartilage
in avascular areas (Figure 6D) in some cases.

Chapter 7

NERVOUS SYSTEM

## I. GENERAL HISTOLOGY

Neuroanatomy and neuropathology are extraordinarily complex subjects which can only be touched upon for the purposes of this book. The reader is referred to textbooks and manuals of neurology for the innumerable details of the extremely complex organization of the nervous system. This chapter contains only certain selected general features and details of basic importance to available information on radiation histopathology and a general discussion of fundamental pathogenesis of radiation-induced lesions of the nervous system.

Generally and basically, the mammalian nervous system is composed of the central nervous system, i.e., brain and spinal cord (Figure 1), and the peripheral nervous system, i.e., the voluntary and sympathetic or autonomic nerves extending from the central nervous system to peripheral ganglia and nerve terminals or endings in body tissues. The cell bodies of the definitive parenchymal cells of the nervous system, the neurons, are largely in the gray matter of the brain (cortex) and of the spinal cord (medulla). The white matter of the central nervous system consists of myelinated axons of the neurons and is predominant in the medullary portions of the brain and the cortical parts of the spinal cord.

The neurons carry out the specialized functions of the nervous system. The main supporting elements of the nervous system are the neuroglia or glia (largely in the central nervous system), the vasculature, and the connective tissues surrounding the various parts of the nervous system. The term neuroglia or glia refers to several interstitial tissues of the nervous system, including: (1) the ependyma, an epithelial membrane lining the ventricles of the brain and spinal cord; (2) the neuroglia proper, consisting of the neuroglial cells (astrocytes, oligodendrocytes, and microgliocytes) and their plasmatic expansions or fibers, which bind the neurons in the central nervous system and in the retina; and (3) the capsular or satellite cells of the peripheral ganglia. The Schwann cells, forming the sheath of Schwann around the peripheral nerves, are homologous to neuroglial cells of the central nervous system.

The neuron usually has a large cell body with a large nucleus and abundant perinuclear cytoplasm. The cell body sends out cytoplasmic processes, usually including several short dendrites and one axon or axis cylinder. The axon varies greatly in length. There are numerous variations in neurons with respect to different combinations of size, shape, position, synaptic relationships, and the variations in the number, length, thickness, and manner of branching of the cytoplasmic processes. Although the neurons are more or less individually independent structurally and functionally, they are related by their synapses with other neurons and their endings with epithelial, muscular, or glandular cells. The axons of some neurons may be long and become peripheral nerve fibers which terminate at a great distance in some other part of the body, while the axons of other neurons may be relatively short and confined to the gray matter containing their cell bodies.

Nerve fibers are axons with coverings of ectodermal origin. In the peripheral nervous system, all axons are surrounded by a neurolemma composed of Schwann cells. There are no Schwann cells around axons in the central nervous system, but homologous neuroglial cells are distributed along the fiber tracts. By light microscopy, all but the smallest axons are surrounded by a myelin sheath. The myelin sheath is regarded as having been laid down and maintained by the cells of the sheath of Schwann in the

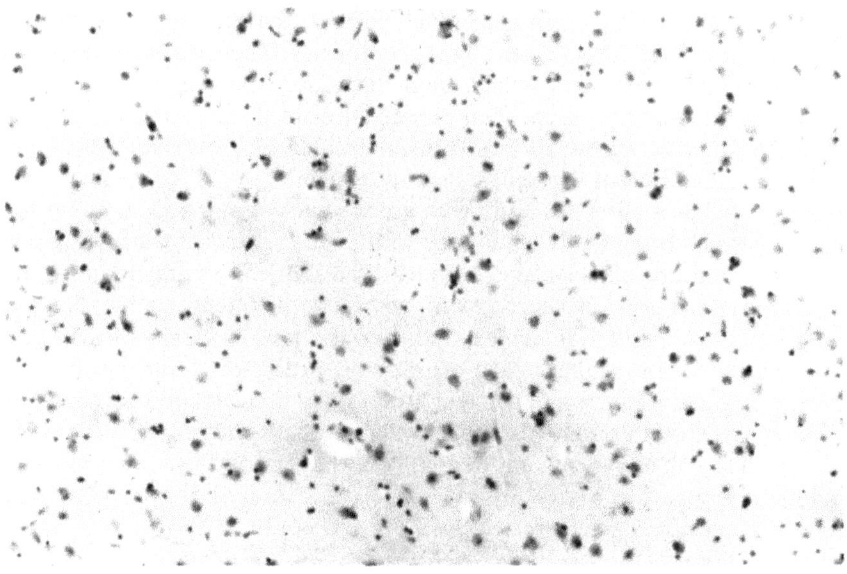

FIGURE 1B.    Rat brain cortex (silver, Alcian blue, periodic acid Schiff stains; approximately 1000×), distinguishing the fine vasculature.

FIGURE 1.    Sections of normal central nervous system tissues. A. Dog brain cortex (H. and E. stains; approximately 750×), showing neuron cell bodies (larger nuclei), glial cells, and fine vasculature.

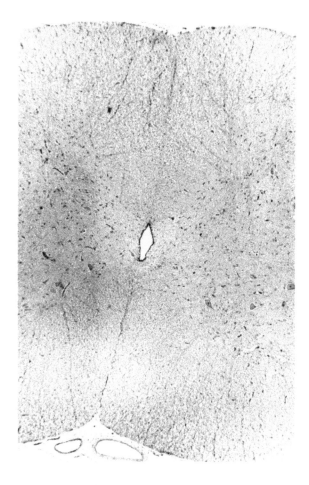

FIGURE 1C.   Rabbit spinal cord (H. and E. stains; approximately 200×).

case of peripheral nerves, or by homologous neuroglial cells in the central nervous system. Since even the smallest visible fibers may show some birefringent material around them under the polarizing microscope, it is possible that all fibers have some myelin around them. The refractility of myelin gives the white color to the fiber masses in the central nervous system and many peripheral nerves.

Schwann cells may be regarded as neuroglial cells extending from the central nervous system as peripheral axons grew. Many of the nerve fibers in the brain and spinal cord, especially those in the white substance, are enveloped not only by myelin sheaths but also by neuroglia, particularly oligodendroglia, instead of a neurolemma. Schwann cells are necessary to the life and function of the axons of the peripheral nervous system. Regeneration of an axon begins in the proximal cut end of an axon and proceeds in the wake of the pathway formed by the Schwann cells.

Of the three types of neuroglial cells proper, the two large types (macroglia), astrocytes and olidodendrocytes, are of ectodermal origin, as are the neurons. The small type (microglial cells) originate from mesodermal cells of the pia mater which migrate into the central nervous system along with the blood vessels. Protoplasmic astrocytes (abundant cytoplasm and numerous thick plasmatic processes), found mainly in the gray substance, are attached to the blood vessels and the pia mater, and some are satellites of neuron cell bodies. The fibrous astrocytes, found mainly in the white sub-

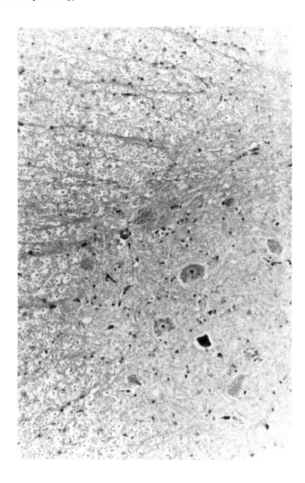

FIGURE 1D.    Higher magnification (approximately 750×) of part of spinal cord shown in C, showing inner gray matter (central right) and outer white matter elsewhere. (A, C, and D from Bradley, E. W., Zook, B. C., and Casarett, G. W., unpublished photomicrographs; B from Eddy, H. A. and Casarett, G. W., unpublished.)

stance, are also often attached to the blood vessel by their thin smooth processes. The oligodendrocytes are generally smaller, with fewer and thinner processes, and not true neuroglia. Because they are closely associated with nerve fibers and often form rows or columns along them, they are regarded as the central nervous system homologue of the neurolemmal Schwann cells in the peripheral nervous system. Oligodendrocytes close to neuron cell bodies are called satellites. The microglial cells have small nuclei and little cytoplasm, with few and short plasmatic processes, and are distributed diffusely throughout the brain and spinal cord. These cells are probably of mesodermal origin. They can assume a great variety of forms, migrate actively, and perform phagocytic functions.

The neuroglial tissues constitute a complicated supporting framework in which neuron cell bodies and their processes are insulated from one another, except at synapse points. These tissues appear to be important mediators for the normal metabolism of the neurons. Also, the surrounding neuroglial elements always react in some way when neurons are affected by local or remote pathologic processes, and are actively involved in the degeneration and regeneration of nerve fibers and in disorders of the vasculature. The neuroglial cells and the Schwann cells are less specialized than the neurons, and under certain pathologic conditions can proliferate rapidly.

The central nervous system contains blood vessels and is enclosed by membranes (dura mater, arachnoid, and pia mater) or meninges composed chiefly of connective tissue. The dura mater and pia mater contain blood vessels. Most of the blood supply to the central nervous system comes from the highly vascular pia mater.

The dense network of arteries in the spinal pia mater provide many small central arteries to the gray substance, some of which provide smaller peripheral branches to the white substance along the circumference of the cord. The capillaries in the gray substance are much more numerous and dense than in the white substance. The many veins leaving the cord form a diffuse venous plexus in the pia mater.

The arteries of the brain are mainly branches derived from the carotid arteries and the large arteries at the base of the brain (mainly the basilar artery and the circle of Willis). Most of these branches run upward in the pia mater before they provide smaller branches to the brain. These small arteries have been regarded as end arteries, with insufficient anastomosis to establish an effective collateral circulation. As in the spinal cord, the capillary supply to the gray matter of the brain is greater than that of the cerebral white matter.

As the central nervous system contains no lymphatic vessels, the cerebrospinal fluid is derived from the capillaries by diffusion through tissue and perivascular spaces which open into the subarachnoid spaces.

Opinions differ as to the location of the hematoencephalic or blood-brain barrier, with various views holding that this barrier is either at the capillary endothelium, at the membrane formed by the processes of neuroglial cells attached to vessel walls, or at the specialized ependymal regions. Some authors have suggested that this barrier comprises a succession of these structures with various thresholds. The choroid plexus is often considered separately as the barrier between the blood and the cerebrospinal fluid.

Before considering the effects of radiation on the nervous system, some consideration should be given to some of the visible changes which occur in neurons as a result of normal physiologic activity or certain pathologic conditions. The chromophil substance (Nissl substance) of the cytoplasm is especially sensitive to normal fatigue and artificial nerve stimulation, when some of this substance may disintegrate into granules or dissolve (chromatolysis), and there may be an associated increase in cell body volume due to increased water content. With extreme fatigue, the chromophil substance may disappear completely and the cell body volume may decrease. After rest, this substance may reappear, unless the fatigue has been too great or prolonged, in which case the neuron may degenerate further and die. Most of the changes in the neuron cell body in fatigue and in various pathologic conditions take the form of chromatolysis, with variations in detail. In the so-called retrograde cell degeneration (axon reaction) which occurs in the neuron cell body after severing of the axon, the cell body increases in size, chromatolysis occurs, and the nucleus becomes eccentrically located in the cell body and may become reduced in size or show shrivelling of the nuclear membrane. The severity of this reaction depends upon the type of neuron, the nature of the damage, the distance between the point of axon interruption and the cell body, and the rate and degree of regeneration following the damage. In other words, the reaction may be followed by complete recovery, partial recovery, or death of the neuron, depending upon these factors. It is thought that neurons in the brain probably always degenerate and disappear completely when their axons are interrupted. The myelinated fibers of neurons whose cell bodies have been destroyed, or which have been separated from their cell bodies, degenerate and their myelin is gradually resorbed. The distal part of a severed nerve degenerates, while the proximal part that is continuous with the cell bodies may change little. Regeneration may restore peripheral nerves.

## II. RADIOSENSITIVITY

Unlike their primitive and proliferating embryonic precursor cells, the neurons are highly specialized, long-lived cells which have lost their ability to divide mitotically under any circumstances (fixed postmitotic cells) and are irreplaceable. The neurons are highly resistant to the direct cytocidal actions of radiation. The Schwann cells of mature nerves, unlike the actively proliferating Schwann cells of developing nerves, are long-lived, highly specialized cells which rarely divide under normal conditions, but which can proliferate under pathologic conditions of nerve damage (reverting postmitotic cells). They are relatively radioresistant. The neuroglial cells of the mature central nervous system, unlike the actively proliferating neuroglial cells of the developing system, also behave essentially as reverting postmitotic cells, in that they normally divide infrequently but may proliferate rapidly for a time in response to tissue damage, and are relatively resistant to the direct cytocidal actions of radiation. Nerve axon fibers are extremely resistant to the direct destructive action of radiation. Myelin also seems to be resistant to direct effects of radiation. Electron microscopic observations that the myelin sheath is composed of layers spirally wrapped around the axon, and that suggest that the myelin sheath is not secreted but is part of the sheath cell, would suggest that changes in myelin may indicate changes in the cells themselves.

Despite the radioresistance of mature neurons and neuroglial cells to the direct destructive effects of radiation, radiation may presumably impair the functions of some of these cells and, in the case of the neuroglial cells, may induce reproductive sterilization in some of them. The small number of neuroglial cells which may be occasionally in cell reproduction may be relatively radiosensitive.

The developing nervous system of embryos and young animals is highly radiosensitive because the actively proliferating and developing primitive neuron precursors and neuroglial cells are relatively sensitive to the direct cytocidal actions of radiation. The radioresistance of the nervous system and its cellular elements increases greatly as maturation is completed. For a given interval after irradiation it takes a larger dose, or for a given dose it takes a longer time, to produce given degrees of nervous system damage in mature animals than in young developing animals.

## III. RADIATION HISTOPATHOLOGY OF CENTRAL NERVOUS SYSTEM

In the mature central nervous system, with its relatively radioresistant parenchymal cells (neurons) and neuroglial cells, the radiation doses required to cause early destruction of many of these cells are very large (many thousands of rads). Inevitably such doses also cause early (within a few days to a week) severe damage to the fine vasculature, with marked congestion, impairment of circulation, increased permeability of vessels and extravasation, disruption of capillary-astrocyte blood brain barriers, perivascular and interstitial edema and acute inflammation, with infiltration by polymorphonuclear granulocytes. With these very large doses there may also be petechial or larger hemorrhages and thrombi in fine vasculature. The early effects on neurons and their neuroglial cells are largely secondary to the vascular damage and its early consequences, with the relatively diffuse effects on cells being secondary to the early diffuse edema and acute inflammation, and with the more localized effects on cells being secondary to the more localized occlusion of arterioles and obstruction of blood flow.

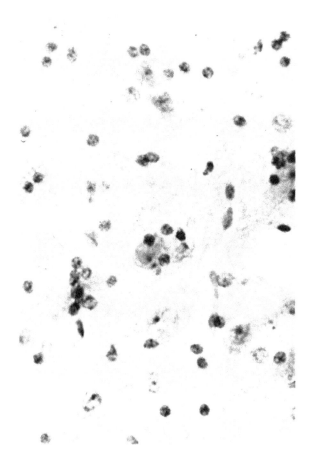

FIGURE 2. Sections of dog brains 63 or 74 days after 3000 rads neutron irradiation. A. Section of gray matter (approximately 3000×), showing small area with a degenerating, congested blood vessel (center) surrounded by edematous tissue containing tiny foci of proliferating glial cells.

The edema causes spatial separation of neuron cell bodies and their processes (axons and dendrites) and neuroglial cells, irregularity of cellular organization, chromatolysis of neuron cell bodies, and degeneration or necrosis of some neurons and neuroglial cells.

The early edema and acute inflammation also develop after moderate radiation doses, but less severely because of the less extensive and more segmentally distributed vascular damage to capillaries and with less acute occlusion of arterioles, with less degeneration or necrosis of neurons and neuroglial cells.

The later chronic and delayed damage in the irradiated central nervous system involves the gradual development and progression of degenerative, necrotic, and occlusive changes in capillaries and arterioles, congestion and hemorrhages, continued edema, and eventual thickening of vessel walls with narrowing of lumens, with secondary chromatolysis, degeneration or necrosis in some of the dependent neurons and neuroglial cells and demyelinative lesions in the white matter, in brain (Figures 2 to 4) and in spinal cord (Figure 5). The degree of such chronic or delayed lesions is directly dependent on dose size, but is also strongly dependent on time after irradiation (i.e., rate of progression of the vascular changes) such that for effective doses, moderate

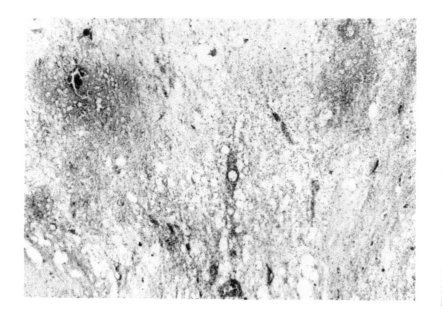

FIGURE 2C.   Section of white matter of brain stem (approximately 750×) showing marked myelopathy consisting mainly of demyelination and axonal degeneration associated with degenerative and proliferative changes in arterioles and other fine vasculature.

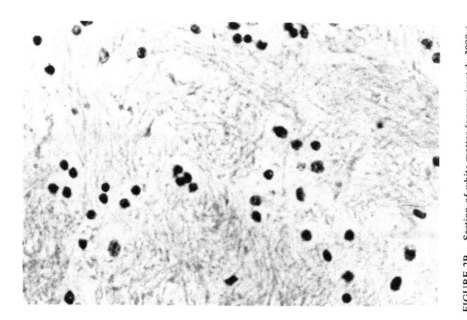

FIGURE 2B.   Section of white matter (approximately 3000×) near gray matter, showing moderate edema and increase in number of glial cells.

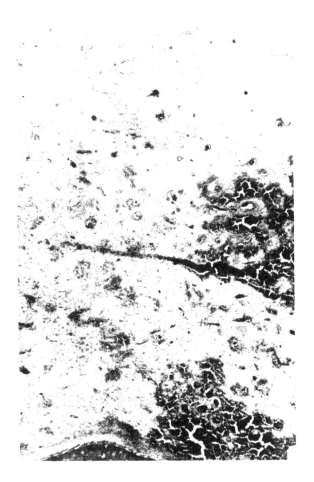

FIGURE 2D.   Section of white matter (approximately 750×)
showing marked myelopathy and hemorrhages associated with
vascular damage and engorgement. (H. and E. stains.) (From
Bradley, E. W., Zook, B. C., and Casarett, G. W., unpublished photomicrographs).

doses can cause similar degrees, but later than at higher doses. Once necrosis of nervous tissue has developed, it may in turn cause acute changes in previously less affected
vasculature, so that delayed radionecrosis of the brain or spinal cord may sometimes
be seen in association with consequences of both chronic and acute vascular damage.
Necrosis and loss of central nervous system cells may be followed by proliferation of
glial cells in a process (gliosis) analogous to replacement fibrosis in other organs.

   The white matter of the central nervous system appears to be much more susceptible
to radionecrosis than the gray matter. In the brain, the brain stem seems to be the
most susceptible region. The most prominent feature of radionecrosis of the white
matter is demyelination, which is closely associated with impairment of oliogodendrocytes, vascular changes, and their consequences. A potential explanation for the differences between gray and white matter in susceptibility to impairment by vascular and
circulatory changes, aside from potentially inherent differences in susceptibility between cellular elements, may be the much greater vascularization and/or astrocytic
barriers in the gray matter. Possibly a similar explanation could apply to the gray
matter of the cerebellar cortex, which is similar in susceptibility to the white matter
and less susceptible than cerebral gray matter.

   The radiation-induced demyelination in white matter is variable in degree and may

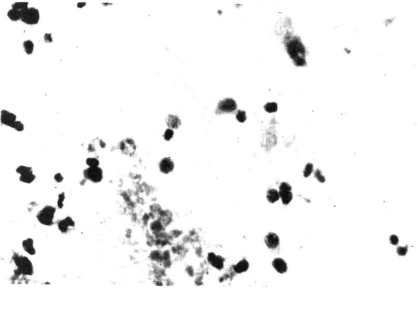

FIGURE 3B. Section from gray matter near white matter (approximately 3000×) showing focal hemorrhage (upper left) and markedly edematous tissue with degeneration and loss of neuron cells bodies elsewhere.

FIGURE 3. Sections of dog brains 74 to 105 days after neutron irradiation (2000 to 4500 rads). A. Section of gray matter near white matter (approximately 3000×) showing focus of necrotic debris from excessively numerous glial cells and some neurons in edematous tissue.

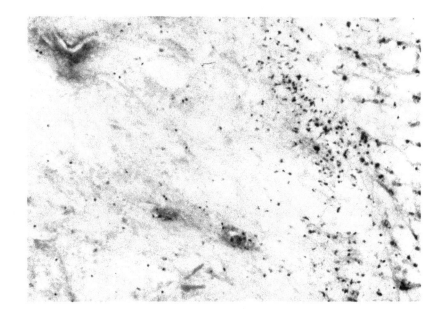

FIGURE 3D. Section of white matter showing severe demyelination and degeneration and loss of axons associated with marked vascular damage. (H. and E. stains.) (From Bradley, E. W., Zook, B. C., and Casarett, G. W., unpublished photomicrographs).

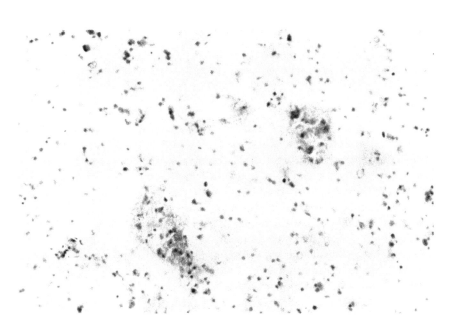

FIGURE 3C. Section of white matter near gray matter (approximately 750×) showing markedly congested blood vessels, edema, and variable demyelination in the area.

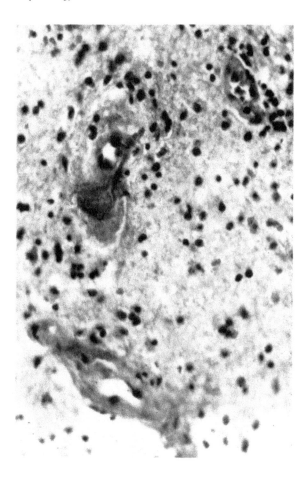

FIGURE 4. Sections of human brain about seven years after approximately 5000 rads focal X-irradiation. A. Marked vascular sclerosis and moderately marked gliosis (approximately 2000×).

be temporary or biphasic, or progressive and irreversible, depending upon the dose. The time after irradiation before demyelination begins to become apparent depends considerably on the natural rate of turnover of the myelin, which is slow enough to permit persistence of the myelin and preservation of the morphologic structures for weeks or months after impairment of the oligodendrocytes. The impairment of oliogodendrocytes probably interferes with the turnover and synthesis of new myelin, but the degeneration of the myelin sheath becomes substantial only after a considerable period of time, and then only if the damage to the cells was great enough to prevent early cell recovery and reversal of the demyelinating process. Temporary impairment of oliogodencrocytes by direct radiation effects and indirectly through the early capillary damage, edema, and inflammation may lead to an early transient myelopathy. This is in contrast to the persistent and progressive myelopathy or delayed myelopathy caused by larger doses.

All types of neuroglial cells show degenerative changes and reduction in number during the acute phase of radiation effect, most prominently the astroglia, similarly but less prominently the oliogodendrocytes, and least prominently the microglia. There is also prolonged inhibition of the glial regenerative processes, partly as a result of direct radiation effects on cells, but to a large degree because of impaired circulation

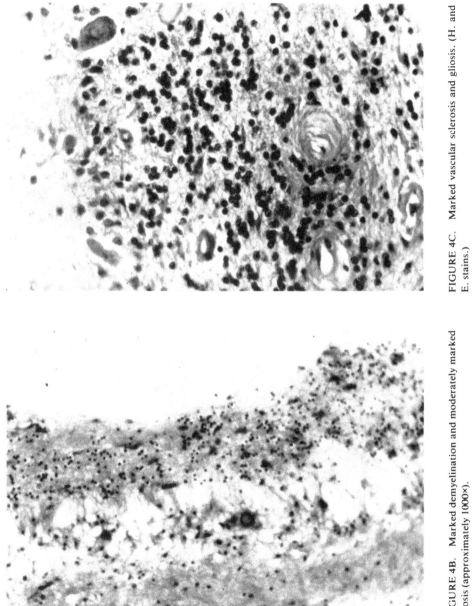

FIGURE 4C.  Marked vascular sclerosis and gliosis. (H. and E. stains.)

FIGURE 4B.  Marked demyelination and moderately marked gliosis (approximately 1000×).

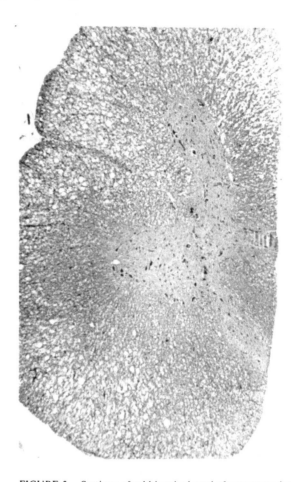

FIGURE 5.   Sections of rabbit spinal cord after neutron irradiation. A. Section (approximately 200×) 17 months after 2520
rads, showing moderately marked demyelination in the white
matter (compare with Figure 1C), with little change in gray
matter (center).

as well. Earlier recovery of glial proliferative activity is observed in regions of neovascularization.

As the proliferation of astrocytes and microglia has been observed in many acute
demyelinating diseases, it has been regarded as a nonspecific effect secondary to severe
demyelination. The demyelination process after irradiation is similar to that in acute
multiple sclerosis.

Some investigators have suggested the possibility that radiation induction of demyelination might involve an allergic or autoimmune mechanism, possibly through damage
of the oliogodendrocyte-myelin complex, with the formation of antigenic metabolites
capable of eliciting either local accumulation of plasma cells and production of antibodies or increase in systemic antibodies. According to Lampert,[335] an antigen-antibody reaction presumably could take place either without a preceding destruction of
the blood brain barrier or only after the vessels had become permeable to antibodies
at sites of vascular damage. In the latter case, the radiation damage of blood vessels
could influence the localization of such reactions. These authors also pointed out that
amyloid has also been found in the irradiated degenerated brain, localized to the perivascular spaces and in the vessel walls, and that one theory has suggested that amyloid
represents the precipitate of proteins active in an antigen-antibody reaction.

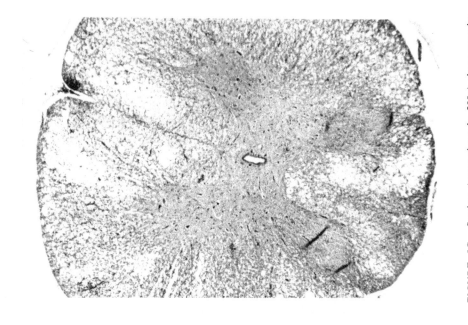

FIGURE 5C. Section (approximately 200×) three months after 3360 rads, showing marked demyelination in the white matter.

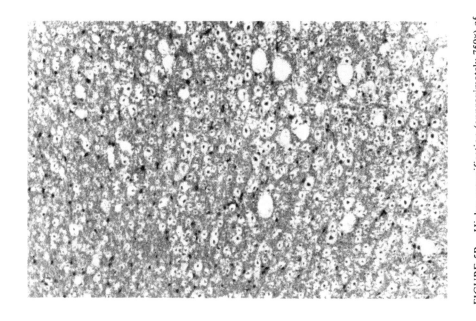

FIGURE 5B. Higher magnification (approximately 750×) of part of section shown in A.

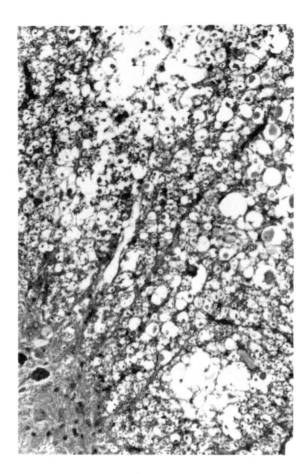

FIGURE 5D.    Higher magnification of part of section in C,
showing demyelination and foci of degeneration and loss of
axons. (H. and E. stains.) (From Bradley, E. W., Zook, B. C.,
and Casarett, G. W., unpublished photomicrographs.)

Degeneration of neuron cell bodies after irradiation, excepting perhaps transient chromatolysis, is not permanent in the early phases of radiation reaction, but may be more permanent and lead to neuron destruction later in the nonselective necrosis of nervous tissue secondary to discrete occlusive vascular lesions.

Careful consideration should be given to investigations directed specifically toward the clarification of the significance of early vascular and circulatory events in the pathogenesis of radionecrosis of the central nervous system, such as the semiquantitative study by Larsson,[336] who found that the first effect of large doses of proton irradiation of the brain of the rat was impairment of the function of blood vessels. This reaction was dose-dependent with respect to earliness of detection and degree at given times, and increased in degree with time. The mild degree or phase was characterized by decreased rate of blood flow in the capillaries. The moderate degree or phase consisted of severe functional disturbances of many capillaries (dilatation, diapedesis, perivascular hemorrhage, aggregates of erythrocytes remaining after perfusion). The marked degree or phase consisted of necrosis or loss of most or all of the capillaries.

The second change in the sequence of events was damage of the blood brain barrier (increased permeability to trypan blue), which accompanied or followed the capillary damage and increased in degree with dose and time as the capillary damage did. After this increased permeability had progressed to a moderate or marked degree along with the capillary impairment, degenerative changes in nerve cells (glial cells and neurons) began to appear, with subsequent progressive degeneration of myelin sheaths and axons, and eventually frank necrotic lesions of varying degrees. These nervous tissue and parenchymal effects were also dose-dependent and increased in degree with time. The mild degree or phase of necrosis consisted of degenerative changes (such as chromatolysis) in many nerve cells or small necrotizing foci of brain tissue. The moderate degree or phase consisted of necrosis of large parts of irradiated brain tissue. The marked degree or phase consisted of general necrosis of most or all of the brain tissue in the path of the beam.

In this study, whenever necrosis was moderate or marked in degree, there were occlusions or necrosis of blood vessels that obstructed the passage of the trypan blue dye, so that the central part of the lesion showed less permeability to the dye and the periphery of the lesions showed marked permeability and intense staining of the tissue. Otherwise no reversal of the changes in permeability was observed.

These observations strongly support the contention that radiation-induced vascular damage is primary to parenchymal damage and may cause most of the parenchymal damage involved in the development of radionecrosis of nervous tissue. However, as indicated earlier, the details of the mechanisms by which vascular damage may cause such lesions at different times after different doses may vary. The early and persistent changes in the capillaries and the blood brain barrier, with the associated increase in resistance to blood flow, erythrocyte aggregation, stasis, edema, inflammation, microthrombi, anoxia or ischemia, may lead to nervous tissue cell damage and eventually to necrotic lesions, as well as to the more slowly developing occlusive lesions in larger blood vessels, but with different distribution of effect and different time intervals.

Rider[344] has reported early demyelinating lesions in the irradiated human brain and spinal cord after a maximum of 5500 R of $^{60}$Co radiation delivered in one month to tumors in the region of the middle ear or jugular bulb. In all cases, the neurological symptoms developed about 10 weeks after irradiation.

Lampert et al.[325] reported a case of disseminated demyelination of the brain occurring about 3 months after $^{60}$Co gamma irradiation (5760 R at 288 R per day) for basal cell carcinoma of the ear. The brain showed intense widespread vasculitis, abundant plasma cells, and areas of demyelination with only slight damage to the nerve cells and axons in the early lesions; degenerative and obliterative alterations of the blood vessels larger than capillaries were present. Jones[333] reported cases of transient myelopathy of the spinal cord in which transient neurologic symptoms became manifest as early as 2 to 37 weeks after irradiation, but found no lesions in the two cases subsequently studied pathologically.

When severe radionecrotic lesions have not recovered by restoration of elements of the original type, the necrotic foci become absorbed in the presence of peripheral neovascularization, fibrosis and gliosis, leaving cysts surrounded by gliosis and fibrosis. The perivascular fibrosis in the region may sometimes be marked, and cortical lesions may sometimes be repaired by the formation of fibrous scars. In the later stages of resolution of severe radionecrotic lesions, cyst formation may be prominent as well as gliovascular lesions. Berg and Lindgren[315] have outlined several different ways by which such cysts appear to develop and grow, namely, by conversion of coagulation necrosis after fibrinoid impregnation of the tissues, by ischemic softening and absorption of the coagulated necrotic tissue, by liquefaction of edematous, loosened, severely damaged tissue without preceding necrosis, and by organization of hemorrhages such as those from telangiectatic vessels.

Boden[316] reported 7 cases of delayed radiation myelitis of the human brain stem, in which the first neurologic symptoms appeared between 11 and 20 months after radiation therapy with total doses ranging from 4500 to 6050 R. The necrotic lesions were circumscribed disseminated placques of demyelination with central necrosis and occasional hemorrhage, and with a wall of microglial cells and marked astrocytic proliferation and plasmatodendrosis immediately surrounding the placques. The vascular changes were marked, with a predominance of degenerative processes over chronic fibrotic processes. The walls of the arterioles, venules, and capillaries showed marked edema and perivascular cuffing with plasma cells and lymphocytes, with fatty and fibrinoid changes in vessel walls.

Arnold et al.[309-311] reported extensive studies of the clinical and pathologic effects of single highly localized doses (375 to 14,000 R) of betatron radiation (23 MeV X-rays) on the brain of subhuman primates up to 24 months after irradiation, using small (1 and 2.5 cm) beams for their long-term studies. This dose range was regarded as equivalent in biological effectiveness to a range of 225 to 8400 R of 400 keV X-rays. They defined the acute stage as 1 day to 6 weeks, the intermediate stage as 6 weeks to 5 months, and the late stages as 5 to 8, 8 to 12, and 12 to 24 months.

Single tissue doses of 7000 R or more (equivalent to 4000 to 8400 R of 400 keV X-rays) caused acute nonselective necrosis of the entire irradiated area, except that the larger blood vessels still remained intact. In the dose range of 5000 to 7000 R (equivalent to 3000 to 4200 R of 400 keV X-rays), the acute pathologic findings were inflammation, edema, hemorrhages, perivascular exudates, disturbances in the white matter, and occasional small areas of acute necrosis. The acute inflammatory responses, edema, and hemorrhages resolved slowly during the following weeks, the damage to the white matter appeared to recover partly, but the areas of necrosis persisted. The majority of the monkeys, upon recovery from their acute neurological syndromes, remained well clinically for a period of four months or longer, after which time there occurred rather abruptly a number of intense and rapidly progressing neurologic disorders as a result of the delayed radionecrosis, followed shortly by death.

In the dose range of 3000 to 5000 R (equivalent to 1800 to 3000 R of 400 keV X-rays), the acute clinical signs usually disappeared within the first week and remained negative until the onset of delayed radionecrosis about six to eight months later. Histologically, the brains of the monkeys sacrificed during the acute stage showed intense inflammation, hemorrhages, exudates, and edema throughout the irradiated part of the brain.

During the intermediate period, histologic study showed only very mild nervous and glial cell changes, but six to eight months after irradiation there was a fulminating course of delayed radionecrosis which was strikingly selective and severe for the white matter, with changes in the cortical neurons being only moderate. However, the neurons of the periventricular and supraoptic nuclei of the hypothalamus were severely damaged. This disintegration of the white matter appeared to begin in part as a demyelinating process and then progressed to actual necrosis of all constituents, including the myelin, axons, and glial cells. There was little reaction around the degenerating areas 5 to 8 months after irradiation in this dosage range. In monkeys that were not irradiated through the brain stem and could therefore survive longer, the areas of radionecrosis within the white matter were slowly becoming filled with glial cells about 10 to 12 months after irradiation, and by 24 months there was marked gliosis of the radionecrotic areas in the white matter.

After doses of 1500 to 3000 R (equivalent to 900 to 1800 R of 400 KeV X-rays), the acute clinical and histologic findings were less severe and shorter in duration. The lowest dose in this range caused moderate inflammation, cerebral edema, and cellular alterations, but no overt neurologic symptoms until after a year or more, when histologic studies showed radiation damage primarily in the brain stem and internal capsule, with moderate changes in the hypothalamus and with some morphological alterations in the cells of the cerebral cortex. Monkeys receiving 750 or 1500 R ($\leqslant$900 R of 400

KeV X-rays) showed delayed radiation effects in the more responsive areas of the brain a year or more after irradiation.

The inverse relationship between the size of the radiation dose and the delay between the time of irradiation and the development of radionecrosis is much more compatible with a pathogenesis of radionecrosis of mature nervous tissue in which progressive vascular damage plays a primary role than with a pathogenesis in which the primary role is played by direct damage to nervous tissue cells.

As Bailey[313] has pointed out, one characteristic of the reaction to radiation in all tissues, the central nervous system being no exception, is the development of degenerative occlusive changes in blood vessels. There is general agreement that alterations in blood vessel walls are found in all phases of radiation reaction in the brain, spinal cord, and meninges. Damage to larger vessels becomes more obvious at longer intervals after radiation and tends to be segmental, so that the number of vessels observed to be so affected in one or several histologic sections gives rise to an underestimation of the number of vessels actually affected. The striking, or more obvious, changes in the walls of the larger vessels are not nearly as widespread in the irradiated area as is the vasculitis involving the smaller vessels in the acute phases of the damage. The occlusion of larger vessels can account for areas of complete infarction in the region of their distribution, but may not account for other affects.

Innes and Carsten[331] have reported delayed effects of localized X-irradiation (3500 R) of the spine on the spinal cord in rats and monkeys. All the experimental animals developed neurologic signs three to nine months after irradiation. Histologically, acute myelomalacia was found in the area of irradiation, affecting the ventrolateral columns but sometimes also the dorsal columns, with the gray matter being left relatively intact. In the damaged regions there was little or no neuroglial reaction.

## IV. THE EYE

The nervous cells of the eye, including those of the retina which contains elements similar to those in the brain and has been regarded as an especially differentiated part of the brain, are also relatively resistant to the direct destructive actions of radiation, but subject to the indirect effects of radiation mediated through vascular damage.

However, as an organ of special sense, the eye is relatively radiosensitive in terms of radiation induction of lenticular opacity which, when progressive and/or severe, may impair vision. The basis for this sensitivity is the radiosensitivity of proliferating cells in the anterior epithelium of the optic lens.

The round biconvex avascular lens of the eye is enveloped by a homogeneous cuticular capsule. Under the capsule, the anterior surface of the lens is a simple layer of epithelial cells, which are relatively flat in the central area and become thicker and arranged in rows toward the equator of the lens, where, in the transitional zone, they become progressively elongated and transformed into lens fibers that migrate to add to the tissue mass of the lens. The nuclei disappear and the outlines of the fibers become irregular and serrated. The fibers are laid down in curved fashion on the surface of the lens, and their ends join at the two poles (anterior and posterior) of the lens to form septal rays from the poles. Fibers are held together and lubricated by thin layers of cementing substance.

In the anterior lens epithelium, the cells in the central area (toward the anterior pole) behave as reverting postmitotic cells or reserve cells. The epithelial cells nearer the equator (preequatorial zone) are engaged in mitotic division regularly under normal conditions and behave as primitive vegetative intermitotic cells, producing daughter cells, some of which differentiate into lens fibers while others remain as vegetative intermitotic cells.

The condition of the epithelial cells and the capsule of the avascular lens is of prime importance to the normal nutrition and metabolism of the lens, as well as the condition of the surrounding medium. The condition of all of these elements depends considerably on the condition of the vasculature of the ciliary processes. New lens fibers are produced continuously throughout life, but the rate of lens growth becomes slower with advancing age. The difference in ages of the lens is reflected in difference in relative proportion of young and old fibers. Excluding cataracts resulting from traumatic injury, known metabolic diseases, congenital defects, etc., there seems to be a process of cataractogenesis related to increasing age. The mechanism is not clear. Although unexplained cataracts may be associated with generalized arteriosclerosis, it is not clear that the degree of arteriosclerosis associated with cataract is generally greater than that in individuals of similar age without cataracts. However, the possibility still remains that degenerative changes in the blood vessels upon which the lens depends may be important in the development of senescent cataract. With advancing age, the lens capsule becomes thicker, more dense, and less permeable. The potential influence of these changes on the metabolism of the lens is obvious, but excess of such changes in cataract cases has not been established.

The primary radiation damage in the pathogenesis of radiation cataract appears to be direct damage of the cells of the anterior lens epithelium. The inhibition of mitosis and the destruction of radiosensitive actively proliferating cells in the pre-equatorial zone of the epithelium temporarily interrupt and interfere with the orderly progression of differentiation and deposition of lens fibers. In addition, radiation appears to interfere with the production and differentiation of normal lens fibers near the equator. Failure of these cells to differentiate and elongate properly, and degeneration of many of them, as they move toward the poles, results in disorganization of the lens bow region. Severe damage or loss of cells in the pre-equatorial germinative zone, that requires repopulation by proliferation of the central reserve epithelial cells (reverting postmitotic cells), some of which are still impaired by radiation damage, may result in incompletely differentiated cells migrating into the lens and undergoing degeneration. Others may differentiate and elongate more normally. The degree and duration of the process of lens fiber disorganization depend upon the degree and extent of the initial epithelial damage and determine the degree of resultant opacity or cataract and whether the opacity will become stationary or progress to severe visual impairment.

Nuclear debris accumulates from degenerate and necrotic epithelial cells and undifferentiated or defective cells and fibers, with the subsequent development of vacuoles in swollen or degenerate lens fibers, or as a result of dissolution of fibers. As lens growth continues, the debris moves from the periphery of the lens at the equator toward the posterior pole of the lens to result eventually in subcapsular lesions and opacities at the posterior pole.

The severity and rate of progression, or the incidence of the progressive type, of radiation cataract are dose-dependent , and the latent period between irradiation and the development of cataract is inversely related to size of the dose. Young, rapidly growing lenses are more susceptible to radiation cataractogenesis than older, more slowly growing lenses. Fractionation of X or gamma radiation doses tends to reduce the cataractogenic effect of the dose and to delay the onset of cataracts. According to the extensive clinical investigations of Merriam and Focht,[340,341] the low-LET radiation exposure doses causing 100% incidence of progressive changes were: (1) for single doses, 700 R; (2) for doses fractionation in three weeks to three months, 1450 R; and (3) for doses fractionated over periods greater than 3 months, 2150 R.

Neutrons are several times more effective in causing cataract than are low-LET radiations.

Chapter 8

# RADIATION SYNDROMES

As is evident from discussions of specific organs in previous chapters, sufficient doses of radiation localized to various vital organs can cause acute, chronic, or delayed damage, and syndromes related to the damaged organs, of sufficient severity to cause death during the periods of acute, chronic, or delayed reactions, depending upon the radiation dose and intensity.

When the whole body is irradiated intensively (e.g., with a single exposure), premature death may result at different times after irradiation (min to years) in association with various syndromes, depending upon the size of the dose. These various syndromes associated with differences in dose size are different by virtue of the differences in the determining organs involved and the time taken for severe damage in these organs to cause death. It should be pointed out, however, that the damage of other than the determining organ in a syndrome may contribute secondarily, qualitatively, or quantitatively, to the syndrome and to death. and its time of occurrence after whole-body irradiation. Such secondary contributions are reflected in the somewhat larger dose to the determining organ required to cause death in the same period of time when certain other parts of the body are shielded from irradiation. Under these circumstances, and also when only part of the determining organ is irradiated, the resulting syndrome and causes of death are not quite the same as after whole-body irradiation, even if the dose used causes death at about the same time as after whole-body irradiation. Generally, however, if the same dose is given under such different conditions of exposure, the survival times tend to be somewhat shorter after whole-body exposure.

Differences in individual susceptibility result in a range of survival times for individuals around the median, mean, or modal survival time for a syndrome. The temporal, order of the succession of closely spaced acute syndromes after whole-body irradiation depends upon the dose and the kinetics of the pathologic changes in the various determining organs. Because of differences in individual susceptibility, individuals may die in the periods of overlap or transition from one syndrome to another and may show a syndrome that combines features of the two. After whole-body irradiation in the lethal range, some individuals may die during one of the earlier acute syndrome periods, whereas others may survive this syndrome only to die later during the period of another syndrome.

In view of these complexities, it is important to qualify the simple and convenient names that have been given to the various acute whole-body irradiation syndromes (central nervous system syndrome, gastrointestinal syndrome, hematopoietic syndrome) in terms of conditions of exposure, survival time, and extent of additional or influential factors, whenever possible.

In this chapter, emphasis will be placed on the prominent syndromes occurring after whole-body irradiation with single doses, with additional general discussion of localized irradiation of the determining organs where feasible. The reader is referred to previous chapters on the specific organs for details of the radiation histopathology in these organs associated with localized organ irradiation.

The prominent acute syndromes after single dose whole-body irradiation, in the order of their occurrence and decreasing threshold dose, are the central nervous system syndrome, the gastrointestinal syndrome, and the hematopoietic syndrome. In addition to these acute syndromes, the delayed effects syndrome associated with life shortening in survivors of the acute syndromes will be discussed in relation to aging phenomena.

In the central nervous system syndrome, the chief determining organ is the brain, the human syndrome threshold is roughly about 2000 rads for man, the syndrome latency is about ¼ to 3 hr for man, the death threshold is roughly about 5000 rads, the death time is roughly within two days, and the characteristic signs and symptoms are apathy, lethargy, tremors, convulsions, ataxia, hypotension, and a secondary shock-like condition; the major underlying determining pathology includes vasculitis, encephalitis, meningitis, and edema of the central nervous system.

Doses above the threshold for the central nervous system syndrome are far above the thresholds for the gastrointestinal and hematopoietic syndromes. Because of temporal differences in development of the fatal functional impairments in the determining organs, the central nervous system syndrome develops during the early part of the latent period for the gastrointestinal syndrome.

For the gastrointestinal syndrome, the chief determining organ is the small intestine, the human syndrome threshold is roughly about 500 rads, the syndrome latency is about three to five days, the death threshold is roughly about 1000 rads, the death time is roughly three days to two weeks, and the characteristic signs and symptoms are malaise, anorexia, nausea, vomiting, diarrhea, gastrointestinal malfunction, fever, dehydration, electrolyte loss, hemoconcentration, and circulatory collapse; the major underlying pathology is depletion of intestinal epithelium, leukopenia, and infection. The gastrointestinal syndrome develops during the latent period for the hematopoietic syndrome, before the full consequences of hematopoietic damage have become manifest in the peripheral blood.

For the hematopoietic syndrome, the chief determining organ is the bone marrow, the human syndrome threshold is roughly about 100 rads, the syndrome latency is about two to three weeks, the death threshold is roughly about 200 rads, the death time is about three weeks to two months, and the characteristic signs and symptoms are malaise, fever, dyspnea on exertion, fatigue, leukopenia, thrombopenia, and purpura; the major underlying pathology is bone marrow atrophy, pancytopenia, infection, hemorrhage, and anemia. The progressive development of leukocytopenia (lymphocytopenia and granulocytopenia), thrombocytopenia, and erythrocytopenia leads to the development of infection, petechial hemorrhages, and ecchymoses, ulceration of mucosal surfaces, and high fever, with a point of crisis in about the fifth or sixth weeks after irradiation.

For intensive whole-body irradiation (low LET) in man, the median acute lethal dose (LD50/60; lethal to 50% of the population within 60 days) has been estimated to be between 300 and 500 rads, and for the LD 100/60 days has been estimated to be roughly in the vicinity of 600 rads. These doses are not known precisely, nor is the influence of age or sex. Deaths in the midlethal range are associated largely with the hematopoietic syndrome, and deaths in the vicinity of the LD100/60 dose involve both the hematopoietic syndrome and the gastrointestinal syndrome.

The delayed effects syndrome in survivors of intense whole-body irradiation is characterized actuarially in experimental animal populations by dose-dependent shortening of the mean life span with a shift of the time-cumulative mortality curve to the left, i.e., to an earlier time scale, without substantial change in the shape of the curve. The diseases and causes of death in the irradiated are generally those to be expected in the population with a normal life span. However, with the temporal shift of the mortality curve to the left after moderate doses, the age-specific incidence of most of these diseases (with some exceptions), especially the incidence of known age-dependent diseases (degenerative and neoplastic), is generally (with some exceptions) shifted to an earlier period in life. The limited studies of physiologic reserve capacity of organs or the whole body of the surviving irradiated animals compared with nonirradiated control animals, at various times after irradiation, have also revealed a temporal shift to the left in the curve of depression of functional capacities in the irradiated populations. In the irradiated animals, there is also a corresponding temporal shift to the left in the curve of the universal degenerative histologic changes (aging-type changes) which develop progressively throughout life in the nonirradiated animals.

A full consideration of the actuarial, pathologic, physiologic, and histologic changes in survivors of whole-body irradiation, in comparison with the manifestations of "normal aging", indicates a strong qualitative resemblance between the progressive and late effects of life-shortening whole-body irradiation and the progressive and late manifestations of aging, i.e., there appears to be premature aging in the irradiated animals.[51] There are some irregular and inconsistent qualitative and quantitative factors which, at present, appear to be exceptions to this generalization and are as yet unexplained, despite a number of possible or plausible reasons. It is likely that the irradiated survivors are a prematurely aged population which also show other radiation-induced abnormalities not related to aging manifestations.

At low doses or low dose rates of radiation, there is a tendency for life shortening to be due virtually solely to increase in tumor incidence rather than to premature nonneoplastic degenerative changes.

Whether or not there is an absolute or practical dose threshold for the life-shortening effect of radiation in populations surviving long after the period of acute radiation effects is not known. Although experimental results of single doses less than 100 rads or so tend to be equivocal in this respect, the probablistic nature of the radiation induction of cancer, associated with theoretical considerations of the mechanisms of this effect at low levels of radiation, leave open the possibility that the life-shortening effect may have no absolute dose threshold.

The principal dysfunction underlying the central nervous system syndrome and resulting death appears to be neuronal functional impairment. The major mechanism of neuronal dysfunction and destruction in the central nervous system syndrome appears to be indirect and mediated through vascular damage, increased capillary permeability, edema, and acute inflammation (vasculitis, encephalitis, myelitis, meningitis, choroid plexitis). Bond et al.[3] cited considerable evidence for the importance of brain edema in a confined space and the resultant increased intracranial pressure in the central nervous system syndrome. Histologic evidence of brain edema is always found, and in several studies concerned with irradiation of the head only, there has been gross evidence of brain edema and increase in cerebrospinal fluid pressure. Furthermore, the acute elevation of intracranial pressure caused by means other than radiation can cause death with signs and symptoms similar to those in the acute central nervous system syndrome caused by radiation. These observations suggest that many aspects of the central nervous system syndrome are results of the edema and swelling of the central nervous system, especially the brain, within a confined space. Bond et al.[3] further suggested that this may help to explain species differences in threshold dose, in that it is possible that the mouse and rat (high threshold doses) may be better able to accomodate such increase in pressure because of their lack of bony fusion of cranial sutures. It has also been observed that cerebellectomized monkeys and guinea pigs and hemidecorticated guinea pigs have tolerated larger radiation doses than nonoperated control animals. With irradiation of part of the brain or head, the doses required to cause the acute central nervous system syndrome and death are usually larger than those required in whole-head or whole-body irradiation.

The principal damage underlying the acute gastrointestinal syndrome after whole-body irradiation is the depletion of the mucosal epithelium of the intestine, with denudation of the mucosal surface, particularly in the small intestine. However, bone marrow damage, especially the resultant granulocytopenia, is also strongly implicated in the signs, symptoms, and cause of the gastrointestinal syndrome after whole-body irradiation. The intestinal epithelial loss results in loss of fluid and electrolytes, malabsorption, nutritional impairment, persistent diarrhea (often bloody), and body weight loss. Both the granulocytopenia and the loss of intestinal epithelium are involved in the occurrence of the infection and bacteremia which occur in the gastrointestinal syndrome after whole-body irradiation. The granulocytopenia has also been suspected of enhancing intestinal cell death and mucosal denudation by infectious microorganisms and perhaps common intestinal bacteria as well.

When less of the active bone marrow is irradiated in the production of the gastrointestinal syndrome, e.g., with irradiation of the gastrointestinal tract in irradiation of the abdomen only, there are lesser degrees of granulocytopenia and infection, the denudation of the intestinal mucosa takes somewhat longer, and the mean survival time tends to be longer than in the case of whole-body irradiation. When only the intestine or part of the intestine is irradiated, these differences are even greater. Also, the median and mean survival times for germ-free animals or for animals treated with antibiotics after irradiation with doses in the gastrointestinal syndrome range are increased considerably as compared with those for ordinary or untreated irradiated animals.

The principal damage underlying the acute hematopoietic syndrome after wholebody irradiation is radiation damage of the bone marrow, although there is probably also considerable contribution from damage to lymphoid organs. The radiation damage to the hematopoietic system results in pancytopenia, with marked reduction in the numbers of various types of blood cells, especially leukocytes (lymphocytes and granulocytes) and platelets within the first few weeks, and later anemia. The granulocytopenia leads to infection, the thrombocytopenia leads to hemorrhage, and the reduction in erythrocyte production, together with a loss of erythrocytes from the circulation by leakage through damaged capillaries and frank hemorrhages secondary to thrombocytopenia, leads to anemia. The period of severe illness is characterized not only by hemorrhage and infection, but also by fluid imbalance, diarrhea (often bloody), and other signs of impairment of gastrointestinal function associated with hemorrhage and agranulocytic ulcerations in the intestines. The relative contributions of the primary and secondary damage of intestinal mucosa in the hematopoietic syndrome are variable and not precisely known.

In regard to the delayed effects syndrome, and "premature aging", Casarett[51] has provided a comprehensive review of facts, hypotheses, and theories. At the histopathologic level, the most important and common radiation-induced effect leading to delayed functional impairment and loss of parenchymal cells of organs after recovery from acute effects, is the progressive reduction in the functional integrity of the microcirculatory apparatus (reduced vascular microcirculation and increased histohematic connective tissue diffusion barrier) caused by an increase in the fibrillar density and amount of connective tissue in and around small blood vessels and interstitially in the parenchyma following in the wake of early damage to the fine vasculature, vasculitis, increased capillary permeability with plasmatic transudation and extravasation, vascular and interstitial edema, and inflammation. This impairment of the microcirculatory apparatus occurs whether or not the organs contain relatively radiosensitive parenchymal cells or have suffered initial temporary or permanent cell reduction. There is good reason to assume that some of the surviving parenchymal, vascular, and connective tissue cells have sustained some degree of one or another kind of irreparable injury of more or less functional significance. However, the time of onset of the delayed parenchymal degeneration appears to depend primarily upon the rate of progression of the changes in the fine vasculature and connective tissue rather than upon the cellular kinetics of the dependent parenchyma. The consequences of the residual defects persisting in parenchymal cells may become manifest when the progressive vasculoconnective tissue damage has reached a degree affecting and placing demands on the parenchyma.

All of these effects of radiation on the cells and tissues of organs are nonspecific for irradiation, i.e., they are not unique for irradiation. The qualitative similarity of the progressive and sequential delayed histopathologic effects in irradiated organs to the progressive histopathologic changes occurring in nonirradiated organs with increasing time or age has been mentioned previously. The similarity of the delayed effects syndrome after whole-body irradiation to the manifestations of premature aging were described generally earlier in this chapter, with respect to the temporal advancement (shift to an earlier time scale) of the cumulative mortality curve, age-specific disease incidence, reductions in physiologic reserve capacity, and histologic deterioration of tissues and organs.

The most fundamental mechanisms (molecular, subcellular, cellular) of the delayed effects of radiation or of the manifestations of aging are not yet established. In attempting to explain the earlier development of the expected diseases and causes of death in a population after life-shortening whole-body irradiation, one has the alternative of assuming that whole-body irradiation induces each of the diseases or causes of death *de novo* in individuals, irrespective of their predisposition, or of regarding such uniformity of response, despite the few apparent and currently unexplained exceptions, as a temporal advancement of the diseases, largely in individuals who would have developed them later, if they had not been irradiated. The latter alternative seems much more plausible. It seems reasonable to view this degree of uniformity of response as evidence that whole-body life-shortening irradiation causes a relatively diffuse, subclinical deterioration of body tissues or tissue components which advances the onset of most, if not all, of the age-dependent diseases to a roughly equal degree.

Although the as yet unknown fundamental mechanisms of the delayed radiation effects syndrome and of aging cannot be compared, their manifestations can be compared in an attempt to determine whether or not there are pathways to disease and death which are common to both.

On the basis of histopathologic and circulatory studies and the results of biochemical studies of connective tissue, in the organs of whole-body irradiated and nonirradiated animals periodically throughout life, in an attempt to compare basic (universal) aging or time changes in tissues as well as contrasting changes, Casarett[42, 51-54, 354-358] proposed the histopathologic theory of aging and of radiation-induced premature aging described below and illustrated diagrammatically in Volume I Chapter 4.

In the normal aging of mammals, the most generalized, universal, and inherent progressive deleterious change seen at the histopathologic level is an increase in the histohematic connective tissue diffusion barrier. This progressive increase in the histohematic barrier involves an increase in the amount of connective tissue and in the fibrillar density and amount of collagenous fibers interstitially and in and around the walls of small blood vessels (arteriolocapillary fibrosis).

The increase in the histohematic barrier leads to decreased functional effectiveness (increased resistance) of the barrier in terms of selective diffusion (microcirculation) of gases, nutrients, and wastes across the barrier. The increased arteriolocapillary fibrosis is associated with the decreased functional effectiveness of the blood microcirculation, even in the occasional instances of hyperplastic neoformation of capillaries stimulated by increase in the histohematic barrier. Eventually the progressive arteriolocapillary fibrosis results in a reduction in the size of vascular lumens, associated with thickened vascular walls, narrowed or obliterated lumens, and reduction in the amount of fine vasculature and microcirculatory function. The progressive increase in degree of these processes with increasing age eventually reaches a point at which the functional inadequacy involved causes a gradual progressive functional impairment and subsequent loss of the dependent parenchymal cells at various rates in various tissues and organs, with resultant progressive increase in susceptibility to stress and infectious disease, development of degenerative disease or neoplasm, and death.

Whole-body irradiation in life-shortening doses advances this increase in vascular change and in the histohematic barrier and their sequential consequences to various degrees in different tissues and organs, beyond those in control animals of the same chronologic age, the degree depending considerably on the nature and radiosensitivities of the cells, tissues, and vasculature of the organs. In irradiated animals, the nonspecific damage to the endothelium of the fine vasculature, and perhaps the interstitial fibroblasts also, by direct and/or indirect mechanisms are the changes of greatest importance among the early radiation injuries in the eventual development of the increase in the histohematic barrier and arteriolocapillary fibrosis which are responsible for the later parenchymal impairment.

# REFERENCES AND OTHER SOURCES

1. **Alper, T., Ed.,** *Cell Survival after Low Doses of Radiation: Theoretical and Clinical Implications,* John Wiley & Sons, London, 1975.

2. **Altman, K. I., Gerber, G. B., and Okada, S.,** *Radiation Biochemistry,* Academic Press, New York, 1970.

3. **Bond, V. P., Fliedner, T. M., and Archambeau, J. O.,** *Mammalian Radiation Lethality. A Disturbance in Cellular Kinetics,* Academic Press, New York, 1965.

4. **Duncan, W. and Nias, A. H. W.,** *Clinical Radiobiology,* Churchill Livingstone, New York, 1977.

5. **Elkind, M. M. and Sinclair, W. K.,** Recovery in X-irradiated mammalian cells, *Curr. Top. Radiat. Res. Q.,* 1, 165, 1965.

6. **Elkind, M. M. and Whitmore, G. F.,** *The Radiobiology of Cultured Mammalian Cells,* Gordon and Breach, New York, 1967.

7. **Friedman, M., Ed.,** *The Biological and Clinical Basis of Radiosensitivity,* Charles C Thomas, Springfield, Ill, 1974.

8. **Gibbs, S. J. and Casarett, G. W.,** Influences of a circadian rhythm and mitotic delay from tritiated thymidine in cytokinetic studies in hamster cheek pouch epithelium, *Radiat. Res.,* 40, 588, 1969.

9. **Gibbs, S. J. and Casarett, G. W.,** Cytokinetic effects of repeated X-irradiation in vivo in the presence of a circadian rhythm in mitotic activity, *Radiat. Res.,* 48, 265, 1971.

10. **Gray, L. H., Conger, A. D., Ebert, M., Hornsey, S., and Scott, O. C. A.,** The concentrations of oxygen dissolved in tissues at the time of irradiation as a factor in radiotherapy, *Br. J. Radiol.,* 26, 638, 1953.

11. **Hall, E. J.,** *Radiobiology for the Radiologist,* Harper & Row, London, 1973.

12. International Commission on Radiological Protection (ICRP), *ICRP Pub. 26,* Pergamon Press, Oxford, 1977.

13. **Kellerer, A. M. and Rossi, H. H.,** RBE and the primary mechanisms of radiation action, *Radiat. Res.,* 47, 15, 1971.

14. **Kellerer, A. M. and Rossi, H. H.,** The theory of dual radiation action, *Curr. Top. Radiat. Res. Q.,* 8, 85, 1972.

15. **Lajtha, L. G. and Oliver, R.,** Cell population kinetics following different regimes of irradiation, *Br. J. Radiol.,* 35, 131, 1962.

16. **Lea, D. E.,** *Actions of Radiation on Living Cells,* University Press, Cambridge, 1955.

17. **Meredith, W. J. and Massey, J. B.,** *Fundamental Physics of Radiology,* John Wright, Bristol, 1972.

18. **Puck, T. T. and Marcus, P. I.,** Action of X-rays on mammalian cells, *J. Exp. Med.,* 103, 653, 1956.

19. **Rossi, H. H.,** Microscopic energy distribution in irradiated matter. I. Basic considerations, in *Radiation Dosimetry,* Vol. I, Academic Press, New York, 1967, 43.

20. **Rossi, H. H.,** The effects of small doses of ionizing radiation, *Phys. Med. Biol.,* 15, 255, 1970.

21. **Swallow, A. J.,** *Radiation Chemistry: An Introduction,* Longman, London, 1973.

22. **Terasima, T. and Tolmach, L. J.,** Variations in several responses of Hela cells to X-irradiation during the division cycle, *Biophys. J.,* 3, 11, 1963.

23. **Bender, M. A.,** X-ray induced chromosome aberrations in mamalian cells in vivo and in vitro, in *Immediate and Low Level Effects of Ionizing Radiations,* Buzzati-Traverso, A. B., Ed., Taylor & Francis Ltd., London, 1960, 103.

24. **Berdjis, C. C., Cell,** in *Pathology of Irradiation,* Berdjis, C. C., Ed., Williams & Wilkins Co., Baltimore, 1971, 10.

25. **Casarett, A. P. and Casarett, G. W.,** Histological Investigations of Mechanisms of X-ray Effects on Spermatogenesis in the Rat. I. Introduction, Purpose, Methods and Preliminary Experiments, II. Studies Comparing Effects of Acute and Chronic Irradiation, U.S. Atomic Energy Commission Reports UR-496 and 497, Washington, D.C., 1957.

26. **Casarett, G. W.,** Interactions between cells and tissues following irradiation, in *Radiobiology at the Intra-Cellular Level,* Hennessy, T. G., Ed., Pergamon Press, New York, 1959, 115.

27. **Casarett, G. W.,** Radiation injury, in *Surgery Annual 1972,* Cooper, P. and Nyhus, L., Eds., Appleton-Crofts, New York, 1972, 103.

28. **Evans, H. J.,** Chromosome aberrations induced by ionizing radiations, in *International Review of Cytology,* Bourne, G. H. and Danielli, J. F., Eds., Pergamon Press, New York, 1962, 221, 301.

29. **Hendrickson, F. R. and Hibbs, G. G.,** Radiation effects on cell cycle dynamics, *Radiology,* 83, 131, 1964.

30. **Lajtha, L. C.,** Inhibition of DNA synthesis in relation to cell death, in *Radiation Effects in Physics, Chemistry and Biology,* Ebert, M. and North, H. A., Eds., North-Holland, Amsterdam, 1963, 216.

31. **Montgomery, P. O'B., Karney, D., Reynolds, R. C., and McClendon, D.,** Cellular and subcellular effects of ionizing radiations, *Am. J. Pathol.,* 44, 727, 1964.

32. **Puck, T. T.**, Action of radiation on mammalian cells. III. Relationship between reproductive death and induction of chromosome anomalies by X-irradiation of euploid human cells in vitro, *Proc. Nat. Acad. Sci. U.S.A.*, 44, 772, 1958.

33. **Puck, T. T.**, The action of radiation on mammalian cells, *Am. Nat.*, 94, 95, 1960.

34. **Rubin, P. and Casarett, G. W.**, *Clinical Radiation Pathology*, W. B. Saunders, Philadelphia, 1968.

35. **Sobkowski, F. J. and Casarett, G. W.**, Chromosome Damage and Mitotic Index in X-irradiated Cells, U. S. Atomic Energy Commission Report UR-668, Washington, D.C., 1965.

36. **Till, J. E.**, Quantitative aspects of radiation lethality at the cellular level, *Am. J. Roentgenol.*, 90, 918, 1963.

37. **Warren, S. , Ed.**, Effects of radiation on normal tissues, *Arch. Pathol.*, Vol. 34 and 35, 1942-3.

38. **Goldfeder, A.**, Cell structure and radiosensitivity, *Trans. N. Y. Acad. Sci.*, 26, 215, 1964.

39. **Bergonie, J. and Tribondeau, L.**, Interpretation de quelques resultats de la radiotherapie et assai de fixation d'une technique rationale, *C. R. Acad. Sci.*, 143, 983, 1906.

40. **Bond, V. P. and Sugahara, T., Eds.**, *Comparative Cellular and Species Radiosensitivity*, Igaku Shoin Ltd., Tokyo, 1969.

41. **Casarett, G. W.**, The Effects of Ionizing Radiations From External Sources on Gametogenesis and Fertility in Mammals, U.S. Atomic Energy Commission Report UR-441, Washington, D.C., 1956.

42. **Casarett, G. W.**, Concept and criteria of radiologic aging, in *Cellular Basis And Aetiology of Late Somatic Effects of Ionizing Radiation*, Harris, R. J. C., Ed., Academic Press, London, 1963, 189.

43. **Casarett, G. W.**, Long-term effects of irradiation on sperm production of dogs, in *Effects of Ionizing Radiation on the Reproductive System*, Carlson, W. D. and Gassner, F. X., Eds., Pergamon Press, New York, 1964, 137.

44. **Casarett, G. W.**, Patterns of recovery from large single-dose exposure to radiation, in *Comparative Cellular and Species Radiosensitivity*, Bond, V. P. and Sugahara, T., Eds., Igaku Shoin Ltd., Tokyo, 1969, 42.

45. **Casarett, G. W. and Eddy, H. A.**, Effects of X-irradiation on Spermatogenesis in Dogs, U.S. Atomic Energy Commission Report UR-668, Washington, D.C., 1965.

46. **Casarett, G. W. and Eddy, H. A.**, Fractionation of dose in radiation-induced male sterility, in *Dose Rate in Mammalian Radiation Biology*, Brown, D. G., Cragle, R. G., and Noonan, T. R., Eds., U.S. Atomic Energy Commission, Oak Ridge, 1968, 14.1.

47. **Cowdry, E. V.**, *Textbook of Histology*, 4th ed., Lea & Febiger, Philadelphia, 1950.

48. **Hsu, T. C., Dewey, W. C., and Humphrey, R. M.**, Radiosensitivity of cells of Chinese hamster in vitro in relation to the cell cycle, *Exp. Cell Res.*, 27, 441, 1962.

49. **Tsinga, E. and Casarett, G. W.**, Mitochondria and Radiation Sensitivity of Cells, U.S. Atomic Energy Commission Report UR-666, Washington, D.C., 1965.

50. **Warren, S.**, The histopathology of radiation lesions, *Physiol. Rev.*, 24, 225, 1944.

51. **Casarett, G. W.**, Similarities and contrasts between radiation and time pathology, in *Advances in Gerontological Research* , Vol. 1., Strehler, B., Ed., Academic Press, New York, 1964, 109.

52. **Casarett, G. W.**, Pathological changes after protracted exposure to low dose radiation, in *Late Effects of Radiation*, Fry, R. J. M., Grahn, D., Griem, M. L., and Rust, J. H., Eds., Taylor and Francis Ltd., London, 1970, 85.

53. **Casarett, G. W.**, Aging, in *Frontiers of Radiation Therapy and Oncology*, Vol. 6, Vaeth, J., Ed., S. Karger, Basel, 1972, 479.

54. **Casarett, G. W.**, Basic mechanisms of permanent and delayed radiation pathology, *Cancer*, 37, 1002, 1976.

55. **Eassa, E. and Casarett, G. W.**, Effects of epsilon-amino-n-caproic acid (EACA) on radiation-induced increase in capillary permeability, *Radiology*, 106, 679, 1973.

56. **Ely, J. O., Ross, M. H., Metcalf, R. G., Inda, F. A., Barnett, T. B., and Casarett, G. W.**, Clinical, pathological, and hematological effects of chronic neutron radiation, in *Biological Effects of External Radiation*, Blair, H. A., Ed., McGraw-Hill, New York, 1954.

57. **Rubin, P., Casarett, G. W., and Grise, J.**, The vascular pathophysiology of an irradiated graft, *Am. J. Roentgenol.*, 83, 1097, 1960.

58. **Metcalf, R. G., Inda, F. W., with Barnett, T. B., and Casarett, G. W.**, Pathology in animals subjected to repeated daily exposure to X-rays, in *Biological Effects of External Radiation*, Blair, H. A., Ed., McGraw-Hill, New York, 1954, 268.

59. **Ullrich, R. L. and Casarett, G. W.**, Interrelationship between the early inflammatory response and subsequent fibrosis after radiation exposure, *Radiat. Res.*, 72, 107, 1977.

60. **Van den Brenk, H. A. S.**, The effect of ionizing radiation on capillary sprouting and vascular remodeling in the regenerating repair blastema observed in the rabbit ear chamber, *Am. J. Roentgenol.*, 81, 859, 1959.

61. **White, D. C.**, An Atlas of Radiation Histopathology, Technical Information Center, U.S. Energy Research and Development Administration, Washington, D.C., 1975.

62. **Casarett, G. W.**, Histopathology of Alpha Radiation from Internally Administered Polonium, U.S. Atomic Energy Commission Report UR-201, Washington, D. C., 1952.

63. **Casarett, G. W.**, Pathology of orally administered polonium, in, Metabolism and Biological Effects of an Alpha Emitter Polonium 210, Stannard, J. N. and Casarett, G. W., Eds., *Radiat. Res. Suppl.,* 5, 361, 1964.

64. **Casarett, G. W.**, Pathology and hematology of multiple intravenous doses of polonium, in Metabolism and Biological Effects of an Alpha Emitter Polonium 210, Stannard, J. N. and Casarett, G. W., Eds., *Radiat. Res. Suppl.,* 5, 347, 1964.

65. **Casarett, G. W.**, Pathology of single intravenous doses of polonium, in, Metabolism and Biological Effects of an Alpha Emitter Polonium 210, Stannard, J. N. and Casarett, G. W., Eds., *Radiat. Res. Suppl.,* 5, 246, 1964.

66. **Casarett, G. W.**, Experimental radiation carcinogenesis, in *Progress in Experimental Tumor Research,* Vol. III, Homburger, F., Ed., S. Karger, New York, 1965, 90.

67. **Casarett, G. W.**, Pathogenesis of radionuclide-induced tumors, in *Radionuclide Carcinogenesis,* Sanders, C. L., Busch, R. H., Ballou, J. E., and Mahlum, D. D., Eds., U. S. Atomic Energy Commission, Washington, D.C., 1973, 1.

68. **Casarett, G. W., Metcalf, R. G., and Boyd, G. A.**, Pathology studies on rats injected with polonium, plutonium, and radium, in *Biological Studies with Polonium, Radium and Plutonium,* Fink, R. Ed., McGraw-Hill, New York, 1950, 343.

69. **Casarett, G. W., Tuttle, L. W., and Baxter, R. C.**, Pathology of imbibed strontium-90 in rats and monkeys, in *Some Aspects of Internal Irradiation,* Dougherty, T., Jee, W., Mays, C., and Stover, B., Eds., Pergamon Press, New York, 1962, 329.

70. **Cloutier, R. J., Edwards, C. L., and Snyder, W., Eds.,***Medical Radionuclides, Radiation Dose and Effects,* U.S. Atomic Energy Commission Symp., Series No. 20 (CONF-691212), Washington, D.C., 1970.

71. **Dougherty, T., Jee, W. S. S., Mays, C., and Stover, B., Eds.,** *Some Aspects of Internal Irradiation,* Pergamon Press, New York, 1962.

72. **Hanna, M. G., Jr., Nettesheim, P., and Gilbert, J. R., Eds.,** *Inhalation Carcinogenesis,* U.S. Atomic Energy Commission Symp., Series, No. 18 (CONF-691001), Washington, D.C., 1968.

73. **Hopkins, B. J., Casarett, G. W., Baxter, R. C., and Tuttle, L. W.**, A roentgenographic study of terminal pathological changes in skeletons of strontium-90 treated rats, *Radiat. Res.,* 29, 39, 1966.

74. **Jee, W. S. S.**, Bone-seeking radionuclides and bones, in *Pathology of Irradiation,* Berdjis, C. C., Ed., Williams & Wilkins, Baltimore, 1971, 186.

75. **Looney, W. B.**, Effects of radium in man, *Science,* 127, 630, 1958.

76. **Looney, W. B.**, An investigation of the late clinical findings following thorotrast (thorium dioxide) administration, *Am. J. Roentgenol.,* 83, 163, 1960.

77. **Marks, S. and Bustad, L. K.**, Thyroid neoplasms in sheep fed radioiodine, *J. Natl. Cancer Inst.,* 30, 661, 1963.

78. **Marks, S., George, L. A., and Bustad, L. K.**, Fibrosarcoma involving the thyroid gland of a sheep given I-131 daily, *Cancer,* 10, 587, 1957.

79. **Mays, C. W., Dougherty, T. F., Taylor, G. N., Lloyd, R. D., Stover, B. J., Jee, W. S. S., Christensen, W. R., Dougherty, J. H., and Atherton, D. R.**, Radiation-induced bone cancer in beagles, in *Delayed Effects of Bone-Seeking Radionuclides,* Mays, C. W. et al., Eds., University of Utah Press, Salt Lake City, 1969, 387.

80. **Mays, C., Jee, W. S. S., Lloyd, R., Stover, B., Dougherty, J., and Taylor G., Eds.,** *Delayed Effects of Bone-Seeking Radionuclides,* University of Utah Press, Salt Lake City, 1969.

81. **Metcalf, R. G., Casarett, G. W., and Boyd, G. A.**, Pathology studies on rats injected with polonium, plutonium and radium, in *Biological Studies with Polonium, Radium and Plutonium,* Fink, R. M., Ed., McGraw-Hill, New York, 1950, 257.

82. **Rubin, P., Casarett, G. W., and Farrer, P.**, The effects of intra-articular[198] Au instillations on articular cartilage, *Radiology,* 103, 685, 1972.

83. **Stannard, J. N. and Casarett, G. W., Eds .**, Metabolism and Biological Effects of an Alpha Emitter Polonium 210, *Radiat. Res. Suppl.,* Vol. 5, 1964.

84. **Tuttle, L. W., Baxter, R. C., Hopkins, B. J., and Casarett, G. W.**, The Retention of Strontium-90 in the rat as Influenced by Dose, Age, and Administration Route, U.S. Atomic Energy Commission Report UR-642, Washington, D.C., 1964.

85. **Voegtlin, C. and Hodge, H. C., Eds.,** *The Pharmacology and Toxicology of Uranium Compounds,* Parts I and II, McGraw-Hill , New York, 1949.

86. **Voegtlin, C. and Hodge, H. C., Eds.,** *The Pharmacology and Toxicology of Uranium Compounds,* Parts III and IV, McGraw-Hill, New York, 1953.

87. **Blair, H. A., Ed.,** *Biological Effects of External Radiation,* McGraw-Hill, New York, 1954.

88. **Bloom, W., Ed.,** *Histopathology of Irradiation from External and Internal Sources,* McGraw-Hill, New York, 1948.

89. **Bloom, W. and Fawcett, D. W.,** *A Textbook of Histology,* 8th ed. W. B. Saunders , Philadelphia, 1962.

90. **Cronkite, E. P., Jansen, C. R., Cottier, H., Rai, K., and Sipe, C. R.,** Lymphocyte production measured by extracorporeal irradiation, cannulation, and labeling techniques, *Ann. N.Y. Acad. Sci.,* 113, 566, 1964.

91. **De Bruyn, P. Q. H.,** Lymph node and intestinal lymphatic tissues, *Histopathology of Irradiation from External and Internal Sources,* Bloom, W., Ed., McGraw-Hill, New York, 1948.

92. **Denstad, T.,** The radiosensitivity of the bone marrow, *Acta Radiol.,* 52, 1, 1943.

93. **Dunlap, C. E.,** Effects of radiation on normal tissues. III. Effects of radiation on the blood and the hemopoietic tissues, including the spleen, the thymus and the lymph nodes, *Arch. Pathol.,* 34, 562, 1942.

94. **Engeset, A.,** Irradiation of lymph nodes and vessels; experiments in rats, with reference to cancer therapy, *Acta Radiol. Suppl.,* 229, 5, 1964.

95. International Atomic Energy Agency, *Effects of Ionizing Radiations on the Haemopoietic System,* I.A.E.A., Vienna, 1967.

96. **Jacobson, L. O., Marks, E. K., Robson, M. J., Gaston, E., and Zirkle, R. E.,** The effect of spleen protection on mortality following X-irradiation, *J. Lab. Clin. Med.,* 34, 1538, 1949.

97. **Jacobson, L. O., Marks, E. K., Robson, M. J., Gaston, E., and Zirkle, R. E.,** The role of the spleen in radiation injury and recovery, *J. Lab. Clin. Med.,* 35, 746, 1950.

98. **Jacobson, L. O., Marks, E. K., Simmons, E. L., Hagen, C. W. Jr., and Zirkle, R. E.,** Effects of total body X-irradiation on rabbits. II. Hematological effects, in *Biological Effects of External X and Gamma Radiation,* Zirkle, R. E., Ed., McGraw-Hill, New York, 1954.

99. **Knospe, W. A., Blom, J., and Crosby, W. H.,** Regeneration of locally irradiated bone marrow. I. Dose dependent long-term changes in the rat, with particular emphasis upon vascular and stromal reaction, *Blood,* 28, 398, 1966.

100. **Lawrence, J. S., Dowdy, A. H., and Valentine, W. N.,** Effects of radiation on hemopoiesis, *Radiology,* 51, 400, 1948.

101. **Lehar, T. J., Kiely, J. M., Pease, G. L., and Scanlon, P. W.,** Effect of focal irradiation on human bone marrow, *Am. J. Roentgenol.,* 96, 183, 1966.

102. **Maisin, J., Dunjic, A., and Maisin, J. R.,** Radiation pathology of lymphatic system and thymus, in *Pathology of Irradiation,* Berdjis, C. C., Ed., Williams & Wilkins, Baltimore, 1971.

103. **Proukakis, C. and Lindop, P. J.,** Hematopoietic changes following irradiation, in *Pathology of Irradiation,* Berdjis, C. C., Ed., Williams & Wilkins, Baltimore, 1971, 447.

104. **Suter, G. M.,** Response of Hematopoietic System to X-rays, U.S. Atomic Energy Commission Document MDDC-824, 1947.

105. **Taliaferro, W. H., Taliaferro, L. G., and Jaroslaw, B. N.,** *Radiation and Immune Mechanisms,* Academic Press, New York, 1964.

106. **Trowell, O. A.,** The sensitivity of lymphocytes to ionizing radiation, *J. Pathol. Bact.,* 64, 687, 1952.

107. **Eddy, H. A. and Casarett, G. W.,** Pathology of radiation syndromes in the hamster, in, *Pathology of the Syrian Hamster,* Progress in Experimental Tumor Research, Vol. 16, Homburger, F., Ed., S. Karger, Basel, 1972, 98.

108. **Borak, J.,** The radiation biology of the cutaneous glands, *Radiology,* 27, 651, 1936.

109. **Borak, J.,** Radiation effects on blood vessels, *Radiology,* 38, 718, 1942.

110. **Devik, F.,** A study of the local roentgen reaction on the skin of mice, with special reference to the vascular effects, *Acta Radiol., Suppl.,* 119, 1, 1955.

111. **Geary, J. R., Jr.,** Effect of roentgen rays during various phases of the hair cycle of the albino rat, *Am. J. Anat.,* 91, 51, 1952.

112. **Hurley, J. V., Ham, K. N., and Ryan, G. B.,** The mechanism of the delayed response to X-irradiation of the skin of hairless mice and of rats, *Pathology,* 1, 3, 1969.

113. **Jolles, B. and Harrison, R. G.,** Proteases and the depletion and restoration of skin responsiveness to radiation, *Nature (London),* 205, 920, 1965.

114. **Jolles, B. and Harrison, R. G.,** Enzymic processes and vascular changes in the skin radiation reaction, *Br. J. Radiol.,* 39, 12, 1966.

115. **Jolles, B., Remington, M., and Simon-Reuss, I.,** Indirect radiation effects and diffusible factors in irradiated tissues (stromatex), *Acta Radiol.,* 56, 57, 1961.

116. **Liegner, L. M. and Michaud, N. J.,** Skin and subcutaneous reactions induced by supervoltage irradiation, *Am. J. Roentgenol.,* 85, 533, 1961.

117. **Lushbaugh, C. E. and Hale, D. B.,** Experimental acute radiodermatitis following beta radiation, *Cancer,* 6, 690, 1953.

118. **MacComb, W. S. and Quimby, E. H.,** The rate of recovery of human skin from the effects of hard or soft roentgen rays or gamma rays, *Radiology,* 27, 196, 1936.

119. **Mount, D. and Bruce, W. R.,** Local plasma volume and vascular permeability of rabbit skin after irradiation, *Radiat. Res.,* 23, 430, 1964.

120. **Teloh, H. A., Mason, M. L., and Wheelock, M. C.,** A histopathologic study of radiation injuries of the skin, *Surg. Gynecol. Obstet.,* 90, 335, 1950.

121. **Tessmer, C. F.,** Radiation effects in skin, in *Pathology of Irradiation,* Berdjis, C. C., Ed., Williams & Wilkins, Baltimore, 1971, 146.

122. **Traenkle, H. L.,** A study of late radiation necrosis following therapy of skin cancer, *Arch. Dermatol. & Syphilol.,* 72, 446, 1955.

123. **Wolbach, S. B.,** The pathological history of chronic X-ray dermatitis and early X-ray carcinoma, *J. Med. Res.,* 21, 415, 1909.

124. **Zirkle, R. E., Ed.,** *Biological Effects of External Beta Radiation,* McGraw-Hill, New York, 1951.

125. **Barrow, J. and Tullis, J. L.,** Sequence of cellular responses to injury in mice exposed to 1000 R total-body X-irradiation, *Arch. Pathol.,* 53, 391, 1952.

126. **Brecher, B., Cronkite, E. P., Conard, R. A., and Smith, W. W.,** Gastric lesions in experimental animals following single exposures to ionizing radiation, *Am. J. Pathol.,* 34, 105, 1958.

127. **Casarett, G. W. and Eddy, H. A.,** Effects of radiation on vasculature of intestine, in *Time and Dose Relationships in Radiation Biology as Applied to Radiotherapy,* Bond, V. P., Ed., NCI-AEC Monograph, Brookhaven National Laboratory, Upton, N.Y., 1970, 101.

128. **Eddy, H. A. and Casarett, G. W.,** Intestinal vascular changes in the acute radiation intestinal syndrome, in *Gastrointestinal Radiation Injury,* Sullivan, M. F., Ed., Excerpta Medica Foundation, New York, 1968, 385.

129. **Friedman, N. B.,** Effects of radiation on the gastrointestinal tract, including the salivary glands, the liver, and the pancreas, *Arch. Pathol.,* 34, 749, 1942.

130. **Friedman, N. B.,** Cellular dynamics in the intestinal mucosa: the effect of irradiation on epithelial migration and maturation, *J. Exp. Med.,* 81, 553, 1945.

131. **Friedman, N. B.,** Pathogenesis of intestinal ulcers following irradiation: effects of colostomies and adhesions, *Arch. Pathol.,* 59, 2, 1955.

132. **Goldgraber, M. B., Rubin, C. E., Palmer, W. L., Dobson, R. L., and Massey, B. W.,** The early gastric response to irradiation; a serial biopsy study, *Gastroenterology,* 27, 1, 1954.

133. **Hollaender, A., Ed.,** *Radiation Biology,* Vol. 1, McGraw-Hill, New York, 1954.

134. **Jennings, F. and Arden, A.,** Acute radiation effects in the esophagus, *Arch. Pathol.,* 69, 402, 1960.

135. **Maisin, J., Maisin, J. R., and Dunjic, A.,** The gastrointestinal tract, in *Pathology of Irradiation,* Berdjis, C. C., Ed., Williams & Wilkins, Baltimore, 1971, 296.

136. **Montagna, W. and Wilson, J. W.,** A cytologic study of the intestinal epithelium of the mouse after total-body X-irradiation, *J. Natl. Cancer Inst.,* 15, 1703, 1955.

137. **Quastler, H.,** The nature of intestinal radiation death, *Radiat. Res.,* 4, 303, 1956.

138. **Roswit, B., Malsky, S. J., and Reid, C. B.,** Severe radiation injuries of the stomach, small intestine, colon and rectum, *Am. J. Roentgenol.,* 114, 460, 1972.

139. **Seaman, W. B. and Ackerman, L. V.,** The effect of radiation on the esophagus; a clinical and histological study of the effects produced by the betatron, *Radiology,* 68, 534, 1957.

140. **Sullivan, M. F., Ed.,** *Gastrointestinal Radiation Injury,* Excerpta Medica Foundation, New York, 1968.

141. **Taketa, S. T. and Swift, M. N.,** Delayed intestinal radiation death in the rat, *Radiat. Res.,* 14, 509, 1961.

142. **Trier, J. S. and Browning, T. H.,** Morphological response of the mucosa of human small intestine to X-ray exposure, *J. Clin. Invest.,* 45, 194, 1966.

143. **Warren, S. and Friedman, N. B.,** Pathology and pathological diagnosis of radiation lesions in the gastrointestinal tract, *Am. J. Pathol.,* 18, 499, 1942.

144. **Engelstad, R. B.,** Pulmonary lesions after roentgen and radium irradiation, *Am. J. Roentgenol.,* 43, 676, 1940.

145. **Evans, W. A. and Leucutia, T.,** Intrathoracic changes induced by heavy radiation, *Am. J. Roentgenol.,* 13, 203, 1925.

146. **Fleming, W. H., Szakacs, J. E., and King, E. R.,** The effect of gamma radiation on the fibrinolytic system of dog lung and its modification by certain drugs: relationship to radiation pneumonitis and hyaline membrane formation in lung, *J. Nucl. Med.,* 3, 341, 1962.

147. **Holt, J. A. G.,** The acute radiation pneumonitis syndrome, *J. Coll. Radiol. Aust.,* 8, 40, 1964.

148. **Jennings, F. L. and Arden, A.,** Development of experimental radiation pneumonitis, *Arch. Pathol.,* 71, 437, 1961.

149. **Jennings, F. L. and Arden, A.,** Development of radiation pneumonitis: time and dose factors, *Arch. Pathol.,* 74, 351, 1962.

150. **Kurohara, S. S. and Casarett, G. W.,** Effects of single thoracic X-ray exposure in rats, *Radiat. Res.,* 52, 263, 1972.

151. **Michaelson, S. M., Schreiner, B., Jr., Hansen, C. L., Jr., Quinln, W. J., Odland, L. T., Ingram, M., and Howland, J. W.,** Cardiopulmonary Changes in the Dog Following Exposure to X-rays, U.S. Atomic Energy Commission Report UR-596, Washington, D.C., 1961.

152. **Smith, J. C.,** Radiation pneumonitis: a review, *Am. Rev. Resp. Dis.,* 87, 647, 1963.

153. **Van den Brenk, H. A. S.,** Radiation effects on the pulmonary system, in *Pathology of Irradiation,* Berdjis, C., Ed., Williams & Wilkins Co., Baltimore, 1971, 569.

154. **Warren, S. and Gates, O.,** Effects of radiation on normal tissues, *Arch. Pathol.,* 30, 440, 1940.

155. **Warren, S. and Spencer, J.,** Radiation reaction in the lung, *Am. J. Roentgenol.,* 43, 682, 1940.

156. **Albert, H. J. and Gillenwater, J. Y.,** The consequences of ureteral irradiation with special reference to subsequent ureteral injury, *J. Urol.,* 107, 369, 1972.

157. **Asscher, A. W.,** The delayed effects of renal irradiation, *Clin. Radiol.,* 15, 320, 1964.

158. **Blake, D. D.,** Radiobiologic aspects of the kidney, *Radiol. Clin. N. Am.,* 3, 75, 1965.

159. **Casarett, G. W.,** A Serial Study of Pathological and Hematological Effects of Intravenously Injected Polonium in Rats, U.S. Atomic Energy Commission Report UR-42, Washington, D.C., 1948.

160. **Fisher, E. R. and Hellstrom, H. R.,** Pathogenesis of hypertension and pathologic changes in experimental renal irradiation, *Lab. Invest.,* 19, 530, 1968.

161. **Guttman, P. H. and Kohn, H. I.,** Progressive intercapillay glomerulosclerosis in the mouse, rat and Chinese hamster associated with aging and X-ray exposure, *Am. J. Pathol.,* 37, 293, 1960.

162. **Hartman, F. W.,** Hypertension and kidney lesions produced by X-ray, *Am. J. Pathol.,* 15, 623, 1939.

163. **Hartman, F. W., Bolliger, A., and Doub, H. P.,** Experimental nephritis produced by irradiation, *Am. J. Med. Sci.,* 172, 487, 1926.

164. **Hueper, W. C., Fisher, C. V., de Carvajel-Forero, J., and Thompson, M. R.,** The pathology of experimental roentgencystitis in dogs, *J. Urol.,* 47, 156, 1942.

165. **Lamson, B. G., Billings, M. S., Ewell, L. H., and Bennett, L. R.,** Late effects of total body roentgen irradiation. IV. Hypertension nephrosclerosis in female Wistar rats surviving 1000 R hypoxic total body irradiation, *Arch. Pathol.,* 66, 322, 1958.

166. **Luxton, R. W. and Kunkler, P. B.,** Radiation nephritis, *Acta Radiol.,* 2, 169, 1962.

167. **Madrazo, A., Suzuki, Y., and Churg, J.,** Radiation nephritis: acute changes following high doses of radiation, *Am. J. Pathol.,* 54, 507, 1969.

168. **Madrazo, A., Suzuki, Y., and Churg, J.,** Radiation nephritis: chronic changes after high doses of radiation, *Am. J. Pathol.,* 61, 37, 1970.

169. **Maier, J. G. and Casarett, G. W.,** Pathophysiologic Aspects of Radiation Nephritis in Dogs, U.S. Atomic Energy Commission Report UR-626, Washington, D.C., 1963.

170. **Maier, J. G. and Casarett, G. W.,** Cellular growth and tissue radiosensitivity: tissue studies in vivo and the concept of radiation nephritis, *Trans., N.Y. Acad. Sci.,* Series II, 26, 599, 1964.

171. **Masterson, B. J. and Rutledge, F.,** Irradiation ulcer of the urinary bladder, *Obstet. Gynecol.,* 30, 23, 1967.

172. **Mostofi, F. K. and Berdjis, C. C.,** The kidney, in *Pathology of Irradiation,* Berdjis, C. C., Ed., Williams & Wilkins, Baltimore, 1971, 597.

173. **Page, I. H.,** Production of nephritis in dogs by roentgen rays, *Am. J. Med. Sci.,* 191, 251, 1936.

174. **Redd, B. L.,** Radiation nephritis: review, case report, and animal study, *Am. J. Roentgenol.,* 83, 88, 1960.

175. **Rosen, V. J.,** Radiation pathology of the genitourinary tract, in *Pathology of Irradiation,* Berdjis, C. C., Ed., Williams & Wilkins, Baltimore, 1971, 592.

176. **Upton, A. C. and Furth, J.,** Nephrosclerosis induced in mice by total body irradiation, *Fed. Proc.,* 13, 445, 1954.

177. **Wachholz, B., and Casarett, G. W.,** Radiation hypertension and nephrosclerosis, *Radiat. Res.,* 41, 39, 1970.

178. **Wilson, C., Ledingham, J. M., and Cohen, M.,** Hypertension following X-irradiation of kidneys, *Lancet,* 1, 9, 1958.

179. **Asscher, A. W., Wilson, C., and Anson, S. G.,** Sensitisation of blood vessels to hypertensive damage by X-irradiation, *Lancet,* 1, 580, 1961.

180. **Berdjis, C. C.,** Cardiovascular system and radiation — late effects of X-rays on the arteries of the adult rat, *Strahlentherapie,* 112, 595, 1960.

181. **Berdjis, C. C.,** Cardiovascular system, in *Pathology of Irradiation,* Berdjis, C. C., Ed., Williams & Wilkins, Baltimore, 1971, 377.

182. **Catterall, M.,** The effect of radiation upon the heart, *Br. J. Radiol.,* 33, 159, 1960.

183. **Cohn, K. E., Stewart, J. R., Fajardo, L. F. and Hancock, E. W.,** Heart disease following radiation, *Medicine,* 46, 281, 1967.

184. Fajardo, L. F. and Stewart, J. R., Experimental radiation-induced heart disease. Light microscopic studies, *Am. J. Pathol.*, 59, 299, 1970.

185. Fajardo, L. F. and Stewart, J. R., Capillary injury preceding radiation-induced myocardial fibrosis, *Radiology*, 101, 429, 1971.

186. Gold, H., Production of arteriosclerosis in the rat: effect of X-ray and high fat diet, *Arch. Pathol.*, 71, 268, 1961.

187. Hurst, D. W., Radiation fibrosis of pericardium, with cardiac tamponade, *Can. Med. Assoc. J.*, 81, 377, 1959.

188. Jones, A. and Wedgwood, J., Effects of radiations on the heart, *Br. J. Radiol.*, 33, 138, 1966.

189. Kundel, H. L., The effect of gamma irradiation on the cardiovascular system of the Rhesus monkey, *Radiat. Res.*, 27, 406, 1956.

190. Lamberts, A. B., Initial X-ray effects on the aortic wall and their late consequences, in *Cellular Basis and Aetiology of Late Somatic Effects of Ionizing Radiation*, Harris, R. J. C., Ed., Academic Press, New York, 1962.

191. Leach, J. E. Some of the effects of roentgen irradiation on the cardiovascular system, *Am. J. Roentgenol.*, 50, 616, 1943.

192. Leach, J. E. and Sugiura, K., The effect of high voltage roentgen rays on the heart of adult rats, *Am. J. Roentgenol.*, 41, 414, 1941.

193. Lindsay, S., Kohn, H. I., Dakin, R. L., and Jew, J., Aortic arteriosclerosis in the dog after localized aortic x-irradiation, *Circ. Res.*, 10, 51, 1962.

194. Moss, A. J., Smith, D. W., Michaelson, S., Schreiner, B. F., and Murphy, Q. W., Radiation-induced Acute Myocardial Infarction in the Dog, *U.S. Atomic Energy Commission Report UR-625*, Washington, D.C., 1963.

195. Phillips, S. J., Reid, J. A., and Rugh, R., Electrocardiographic and pathologic changes after cardiac X-irradiation in dogs, *Am. Heart J.*, 68, 524, 1964.

196. Rubin, E., Camara, J., Grayzel, D. M., and Zak, F. G., Radiation-induced cardiac fibrosis, *Am. J. Med.*, 34, 71, 1963.

197. Sams, A., Histological changes in the larger blood vessels of the hind limb of the mouse after X-irradiation, *Int. J. Radiat. Biol.*, 9, 165, 1965.

198. Smith, D. J., Effects of gamma irradiation on isolated surviving arteries and their vasa vasorum, *Am. J. Physiol.*, 201, 901, 1961.

199. Stewart, J. R., Radiation-induced heart disease, *Radiology*, 89, 302, 1967.

200. Stewart, J. R., Cohn, K. E., Fajardo, L. F., Hancock, E. W., and Kaplan, H. S., Radiaion induced heart disease: a study of twenty-five patients, *Radiology*, 89, 303, 1967.

201. Stewart, J. R., Fajardo, L. F., Cohn, K. E., and Page, V., Experimental radiation-induced heart disease in rabbits, *Radiology*, 91, 814, 1968.

202. Warren, S., Effects of radiation on the cardiovascular system, *Arch. Pathol.*, 34, 1079, 1942.

203. Warthin, A. S. and Pohle, E. A., The effect of roentgen rays on the heart. I. The microscopic changes in the heart muscle of rats and rabbits following a single exposure, *J.A.M.A.*, 89, 1925, 1927.

204. Whitfield, A. G. W. and Kunkler, P. B. Radiation reactions in the heart, *Br. Heart J.*, 19, 53, 1957.

205. Cherry, C. P. and Glucksmann, A., Injury and repair following irradiation of salivary glands in male rats, *Br. J. Radiol.*, 32, 596, 1959.

206. English, J. A., Wheatcraft, M. G., Lyon, H. W., and Miller, C., Long-term observations of radiation changes in salivary glands and the general effects of 1,000 R to 1,750 R of X-ray radiation administered to the head of dogs, *Oral Surg. Oral Med. Oral Pathol.*, 8, 87, 1955.

207. Evans, J. C. and Ackerman, L. V., Irradiated and obstructed submaxillary salivary glands simulating cervical lymph node metastasis, *Radiology*, 62, 500, 1954.

208. Frank, R. M., Herdly, J., and Philippe, E., Acquired dental defects and salivary gland lesions after irradiation for carcinomas, *J. Am. Dent. Assoc. Dent Cosmos*, 70, 868, 1965.

209. Glucksmann, A. and Cherry, C. P., Effects of irradiation on salivary glands, in *Pathology of Irradiation*, Berdjis, C. C., Ed., Williams & Wilkins, Baltimore, 1971, 290.

210. Kashima, H. K., Kirkham, W. B., and Andrews, J. R., Postirradiation sialadenitis: a study of the clinical features, histopathologic changes and serum enzyme variations following irradiation of human salivary glands, *Am. J. Roentgenol.*, 94, 271, 1965.

211. Shafer, W. G., The effect of single and fractionated doses of selectively applied X-ray irradiation on the histologic structure of the major salivary glands of the rat, *J. Dent. Res.*, 32, 796, 1953.

212. White, S. C. and Casarett, G. W., Induction of experimental autoallergic sialadenitis, *J. Immunol.*, 12, 178, 1974.

213. White, S. C. and Casarett, G. W., Effects of irradiation on experimental autoallergic sialadenitis, *Radiat. Res.*, 57, 276, 1974.

214. Ariel, I. M., Effect of single massive doses of roentgen radiation upon the liver: experimental study, *Radiology*, 57, 561, 1951.

215. **Bolliger, A. and Inglis, K.,** Experimental liver disease produced by X-ray irradiation of the exposed organ, *J. Pathol. Bacteriol.,* 36, 19, 1933.

216. **Brams, J. and Darnbacker, L.,** The effect of X-rays on the gallbladder: experimental production of an X-ray cholecystitis, *Radiology,* 13, 103, 1929.

217. **Case, J. T. and Warthin, A. S.,** The occurrence of hepatic lesions in patients treated by intensive deep roentgen irradiation, *Am. J. Roentgenol.,* 12, 27, 1924.

218. **Gershbein, L. L.,** X-irradiation and liver regeneration in partially hepatectomized rats, *Am. J. Physiol.,* 185, 245, 1956.

219. **Ingold, J. A., Reed, G. B., Kaplan, H. S., and Bagshaw, M. A.,** Radiation hepatitis, *Am. J. Roentgenol.,* 93, 200, 1965.

220. **Lacassagne, A. M. B.,** The liver, in *Pathology of Irradiation,* Berdjis, C. C., Ed., Williams & Wilkins Co., Baltimore, 1971, 345.

221. **Pohle, E. A. and Bunting, C. H.,** Studies of the effect of roentgen rays on the liver, *Acta Radiol.,* 13, 117, 1932.

222. **Reed, G. B. and Cox, A. J., Jr.,** The human liver after radiation injury, *Am. J. Pathol.,* 48, 597, 1966.

223. **Weinbren, K. and Ghorpade, K. V.,** The effect of bile duct ligation on latent irradiation effects in the rat liver, *Br. J. Radiol.,* 33, 426, 1960.

224. **Weinbren, K., Fitschen, W., and Cohen, M.,** The unmasking by regeneration of latent irradiation effects in the rat liver, *Br. J. Radiol.,* 33, 419, 1960.

225. **White, J. , Corydon, C. C., David, P. W., and Ally, M. S.,** Cirrhosis of the liver in rats following total-body X-irradiation, *J. Natl. Cancer Inst.,* 15, 1155, 1955.

226. **Archambeau, J., Griem, M., and Harper, P.,** The effect of 250kV X-rays on the dog pancreas; morphological and functional changes. *Radiat. Res.,* 28, 243, 1966.

227. **Fisher, N. F., Grott, J. T., and Bachem, A.,** The effect of X-ray on the pancreas, *Am. J. Physiol.,* 76, 299, 1926.

228. **Leven, N. L.,** An experimental study: the effect of radium emanation on the pancreas of dogs, *Am. J. Cancer,* 18, 899, 1933.

229. **Sommers, S. C.,** Effects of irradiation on endocrine glands, in *Pathology of Irradiation,* Berdjis, C. C., Ed., Williams & Wilkins, Baltimore, 1971, 408.

230. **Spalding, J. F. and Lushbaugh, C. C.,** Radiopathology of islets of Langerhans in rats, *Fed. Proc.,* 14, 420, 1955.

231. **Volk, V. W., Wellmann, K. F., and Lewitan, A.,** The effect of irradiation on the fine structure and enzymes of the dog pancreas, *Am. J. Pathol.,* 48, 721, 1966.

232. **Wellmann, K. F., Volk, B. W., and Lewitan, A.,** The effect of radiation on the fine structure and enzyme content of the dog pancreas. II. Long term studies, *Lab. Invest.,* 15, 100, 1966.

233. **Lawrence, J. H., Nelson, W. O., and Wilson, H.,** Roentgen irradiation of the hypophysis, *Radiology,* 29, 446, 1937.

234. **Linfoot, J. A. and Greenwood, F. C.,** Effect of heavy particle pituitary irradiation, *J. Clin. Endocrinol.,* 25, 1515, 1965.

235. **Mateyko, G. M. and Charipper, H. A.,** Histological effects upon pars anterior of rat following hypophyseal cathode ray irradiation and whole-body irradiation, *J. Morphol.,* 93, 533, 1953.

236. **Pourquier, H., Baker, J. R., Giaux, G., and Benirschke, K.,** Localized roentgen-ray beam irradiation of the hypophysohypothalamic region of guinea pigs with a 2 million volt Van de Graaff generator, *Am. J. Roentgenol.,* 80, 840, 1958.

237. **Simpson, M. E., Van Wagenen, G., Van Dyke, D. C., Koneff, A. A., and Tobias, C. A.,** Deuteron irradiation of the monkey pituitary, *Endocrinology,* 65, 831, 1959.

238. **Tobias, C. A., Anger, H. O., and Lawrence, J. H.,** Radiological use of high energy deuterons and alpha particles, *Am. J. Roentgenol.,* 67, 1, 1952.

239. **Van Dyke, D. C., Simpson, M. E., Koneff, A. A., and Tobias, C. A.,** Long-term effects of deuteron irradiation of the rat pituitary, *Endocrinology,* 64, 240, 1959.

240. **Desjardins, A. U.,** Effect of irradiation on suprarenal gland, *Am. J. Roentgenol.,* 19, 453, 1928.

241. **Engelstad, R. B. and Torgersen, O.,** Experimental investigations on effects of roentgen rays on suprarenal glands in rabbits, *Acta Radiol.,* 18, 671, 1937.

242. **Fischer, N. F., Larson, E., and Bachem, A.,** The effect of X-rays on the adrenal glands, *Endocrinology,* 12, 335, 1928.

243. **Kovacsh, L.,** On the morphologic and functional changes in the adrenal cortex by ionizing radiation in supralethal doses, *Strahlentherapie,* 129, 238, 1966.

244. **Leblond, C. P. and Segal, G.,** Differentiation between the direct and indirect effects of roentgen rays upon the organs of normal and adrenalectomized rats, *Am. J. Roentgenol.,* 47, 302, 1942.

245. **Selye, H.,** General adaptation syndrome and diseases of adaptation, *J. Clin. Endocrinol.,* 6, 117, 1946.

246. **Bender, A. E.**, Experimental X-irradiation of the rat thyroid, *Br. J. Radiol.*, 21, 244, 1948.

247. **Bower, J. O. and Clark, J. H.**, The resistance of the thyroid gland to the action of radium rays. The results of experimental implantation of radium needle in the thyroid of dogs, *Am. J. Roentgenol.*, 10, 632, 1923.

248. **Eckert, C. T., Probstein, J. G., and Galinson, S.**, Radiation of the thyroid: an experimental study in radiosensitivity of the thyroid, *Radiology*, 29, 40, 1937.

249. **Einhorn, J. and Wilkholm, G.**, Hypothyroidism after external irradiation to the thyroid region, *Radiology*, 88, 326, 1967.

250. **Findlay, D. and Leblond, C. P.**, Partial destruction of rat thyroid by large doses of radioiodine, *Am. J. Roentgenol.*, 59, 387, 1948.

251. **Goldberg, R. C., Chaikoff, I. L., Lindsay, S., and Feller, D. D.**, Histopathological changes induced in the normal thyroid and other tissues of the rat by internal radiation with various doses of radioactive iodine, *Endocrinology*, 46, 72, 1950.

252. **Goolden, A. W. G. and Davey, J. B.**, The ablation of normal thyroid tissue with iodine-131, *Br. J. Radiol.*, 36, 340, 1963.

253. **Lindsay, S., Dailey, M. E., and Jones, M. D.**, Histologic effects of various types of ionizing radiation on normal and hyperplastic human thyroid glands, *J. Clin. Endocrinol.*, 14, 1179, 1954.

254. **Michaelson, S. M., Quinlan, W., Jr., Casarett, G. W., and Mason, W. B.**, Radiation-induced thyroid dysfunction in the dog, *Radiat. Res.*, 30, 38, 1967.

255. **St. Aubin, P. M., Knisely, R. M., and Andrews, G. A.**, External irradiation of the thyroid gland in dogs: effects of large doses of roentgen rays upon histologic structure and I$^{131}$ metabolism, *Am. J. Roentgenol.*, 78, 864, 1957.

256. **Walters, O. M., Anson, B. J., and Ivy, A. C.**, The effects of X-rays on the thyroid and parathyroid glands, *Radiology*, 16, 52, 1931.

257. **Zimnitzky, B. S., Baskina, N. A., and Devirz, A. P.**, The effect of the X-rays upon the fine structure of the parenchyma of the thyroid gland, *Radiology*, 27, 68, 1936.

258. **Carlson, W. and Gassner, F., Eds.**, *Effects of Ionizing Radiation on the Reproductive System*, Pergamon Press, New York, 1964.

259. **Dunlap, C. E.**, The effect of roentgen rays and exposure to radium on fertility, *Hum. Fertil.*, 12, 33, 1947.

260. **Eschenbrenner, A. B., and Miller, E.**, Effect of roentgen rays on the testis. Quantitative histological analysis following whole body exposure of mice, *Arch. Pathol.*, 50, 736, 1950.

261. **Fogg, L. C. and Cowing, R. F.**, Changes in cell morphology and histochemistry of testis following irradiation and their relation to other induced testicular changes; quantitative random sampling of germinal cells at intervals following direct irradiation, *Cancer Res.*, 11, 23, 1951.

262. **Fogg, L. C. and Cowing, R. F.**, Effect of direct X-irradiation on mammalian testicles, *Exp. Cell Res.*, 3, 19, 1952.

263. **Glucksmann, A.**, The effects of radiation on reproductive organs; certain aspects of the action of radiation on living cells, *Br. J. Radiol. Suppl.*, 1, 101, 1947.

264. **Halberstaedter, T. and Ickowicz, M.**, The early effects of X-rays on the ovaries of the rat, *Radiology*, 48, 369, 1947.

265. **Heller, C. G. and Clermont, Y.**, Spermatogenesis in man: an estimate of its duration, *Science*, 140, 184, 1963.

266. **Heller, M.**, The testis, in *Histopathology of Irradiation from External and Internal Sources*, Bloom, W., Ed., McGraw-Hill, New York, 1948.

267. **Ingram, D. C.**, Fertility and oocyte numbers after X-irradiation of the ovary, *J. Endocrinol.*, 17, 81, 1958.

268. **Lushbaugh, C. C. and Casarett, G. W.**, The effects of gonadal irradiation in clinical radiation therapy. A review, *Cancer*, 37, 1111, 1976.

269. **Mandl, A. M.**, A quantitative study of the sensitivity of oocytes to X-irradiation, *Proc. Roy. Soc. London Ser. B*, 150, 53, 1959.

270. **Mandl, A. M.**, The radiosensitivity of oocytes at different stages of maturation, *Proc. Roy. Soc. London Ser. B.*, 158, 119, 1963.

271. **Mandl, A. M.**, The radiosensitivity of germ cells, *Biol. Rev.*, 39, 288, 371, 1964.

272. **Oakberg, E. F.**, Degeneration of spermatogonia of the mouse following exposure to X-rays and stages in the mitotic cycle at which cell death occurs, *J. Morphol.*, 97, 39, 1961.

273. **Oakberg, E. F. and Clark, E.**, Species comparisons of radiation response of the gonads, in *Effects of Ionizing Radiation on the Reproductive System*, Carlson, W. and Gassner, F., Eds., Pergamon Press, New York, 1964, 11.

274. **Shaver, S. L.**, X-irradiation injury and repair in the germinal epithelium of male rats. I. Injury and repair in adult rats, *Am. J. Anat.*, 92, 391, 1953.

275. **Silini, G., Hornsey, S., and Bewley, D. K.,** Effects of X-ray and neutron dose fractionation on the mouse testis, *Radiat. Res.,* 19, 50, 1963.
276. **Van Wagenen, G. and Gardner, W. U.,** X-irradiation of the ovary in the monkey, *Fertil. & Steril.,* 11, 291, 1960.
277. **Warren, S.,** Effects on the gonads, *Arch. Pathol.,* 35, 124, 1943.
278. **Zuckerman, S.,** The sensitivity of the gonads to radiation, *Clin. Radiol.,* 16, 1, 1965.
279. **Adkins, K. F.,** The effect of single doses of X-radiation on mandibular growth, *Br. J. Radiol.,* 39, 602, 1966.
280. **Barr, E., Lingley, J. R., and Gall, E. A.,** The effect of roentgen irradiation on epiphyseal growth, *Am. J. Roentgenol.,* 49, 104, 1943.
281. **Baserga, R., Lisco, H., and Cater, D. B.,** The delayed effects of external gamma irradiation on the bones of rats, *Am. J. Pathol.,* 39, 455, 1961.
282. **Bensted, J. P. M. and Courtenay, V. D.,** Histological changes in the rat bone after varying doses of X-rays with particular reference to tumor production, *Br. J. Radiol.,* 38, 261, 1965.
283. **Bisgard, J. O. and Hunt, H. B.,** Influence of roentgen rays and radium on epiphyseal growth of long bones, *Radiology,* 26, 56, 1936.
284. **Blackburn, J. and Wells, A. B.,** Radiation damage to growing bone: the effect of X-ray doses of 100-1000R on mouse tibia and knee joint, *Br. J. Radiol.,* 36, 427, 1963.
285. **Bonfiglio, M.,** The pathology of fracture of the femoral neck following irradiation, *Am. J. Roentgenol.,* 70, 449, 1953.
286. **Casarett, G. W., Tuttle, L. W., and Baxter, R. C.,** Pathology of imbibed $^{90}$Sr in rats and monkeys, in *Some Aspects of Internal Irradiation,* Dougherty, T. F., Jee, W. S. S., Mays, C. W., and Stover, B. J., Eds., Pergamon Press, New York, 1962, 329.
287. **Dougherty, T. F., Jee, W. S. S., Mays, C. W., and Stover, B. J., Eds.,** Some Aspects of Internal Irradiation, Pergamon Press, New York, 1962.
288. **Ewing, J.,** Radiation osteitis, *Acta Radiol.,* 6, 399, 1926.
289. **Frantz, C. H.,** Extreme retardation of epiphyseal growth from roentgen irradiation, *Radiology,* 55, 720, 1950.
290. **Gall, E. A., Lingley, J. R., and Hilcken, J. A.,** Comparative experimental studies of 200 kilovolt and 1000 kilovolt roentgen rays. I. The biological effects on the epiphysis of the albino rat, *Am. J. Pathol.,* 16, 605, 1940.
291. **Gates, O.,** Effects of radiation in normal tissues. Effects on bone, cartilage, and teeth., *Arch. Pathol.,* 35, 323, 1943.
292. **Heller, M.,** Bone, in *Histopathology of Irradiation from External and Internal Sources,* Bloom, W., Ed., McGraw-Hill, New York, 1948.
293. **Hinkel, C. L.,** Effect of roentgen rays upon the growing long bones of albino rats. I. Quantitative studies of the growth limitation following irradiation, *Am. J. Roentgenol.,* 47, 439, 1942.
294. **Hinkel, C. L.,** The effect of irradiation upon the composition and vascularity of growing rat bones, *Am. J. Roentgenol.,* 50, 516, 1943.
295. **Hinkel, C. L.,** The effect of roentgen rays upon the growing long bones of albino rats. II. Histopathological changes involving endochondral growth centers, *Am. J. Roentgenol.,* 49, 321, 1943.
296. **Jee, W. S. S.,** Bone-seeking radionuclides and bones, in *Pathology of Irradiation,* Berdjis, C. C., Ed., Williams & Wilkins, Baltimore, 1971, 186.
297. **King, M. A., Casarett, G. W., Weber, D. A., and Burgener, F. A.,** An imaging, autoradiographic, isotopic, and histopathologic study of irradiated bone, *J. Nucl. Med.,* 18, 604, 1977.
298. **Mays, C. W., Jee, W. S. S., Lloyd, R. D., Stover, B. J., Dougherty, J. H., and Taylor, G. N., Eds.,** *Delayed Effects of Bone-Seeking Radionuclides,* University of Utah Press, Salt Lake City, 1969.
299. **Melanotte, P. L. and Follis, R. H.,** Early effects of X-irradiation on cartilage and bone, *Am. J. Pathol.,* 39, 1, 1961.
300. **Neuhauser, E. B., Wittenborg, M. H., Berman, C. Z., and Cohen, J.,** Irradiation effects of roentgen therapy on the growing spine, *Radiology,* 59, 637, 1952.
301. **Ng, E., Chambers, F. W., Jr., Ogden, H. S., Coggs, G. C., and Crane, J. T.,** Osteomyelitis of the mandible following irradiation. An experimental study, *Radiology,* 72, 68, 1959.
302. **Phillips, R. D. and Kimeldorf, D. J.,** Acute and long-term effects of X-irradiation on skeletal growth in the rat, *Am. J. Physiol.,* 207, 1447, 1964.
303. **Reidy, J. A., Lingley, J. R., Gall, E. A., and Barr, J. S.,** The effect of roentgen irradiation on epiphyseal growth. II. Experimental studies upon the dog, *J. Bone J. Surg.,* 29, 853, 1947.
304. **Rubin, P., Andrews, J. R., Swarm, R., and Gump, H.,** Radiation induced dysplasias of bone, *Am. J. Roentgenol.,* 82, 206, 1959.
305. **Vaughan, J.,** The effects of skeletal irradiation, *Clin. Orthop.,* 56, 283, 1968.
306. **Ward, H. W. C.,** Disordered vertebral growth following irradiation, *Br. J. Radiol.,* 38, 459, 1965.

307. Wildermuth, O. and Cantril, S. T., Radiation necrosis of the mandible, *Radiology,* 61, 771, 1957.

308. Young, L. W., Rubin, P., and Casarett, G., Cysteamine protection against irradiation effects on growing cartilage, *Radiology,* 79, 569, 1962.

309. Arnold, A. and Bailey, P., Alterations in the glial cells following irradiation of the brain in primates, *Arch. Pathol.,* 57, 383, 1954.

310. Arnold, A., Bailey, P., and Harvey, R. A., Intolerance of the primate brainstem and hypothalamus to conventional and high energy radiations, *Neurology,* 4, 575, 1954.

311. Arnold, A., Bailey, P., and Laughlin, J. S., Effects of betatron radiations on the brain of primates, *Neurology,* 4, 165, 1954.

312. Asscher, A. W., and Anson, S. G., Arterial hypertension and irradiation damage to the nervous system, *Lancet,* 2, 1343, 1962.

313. Bailey, O. T., Basic problems in the histopathology of radiation of the central nervous system, in *Response of the Nervous System to Ionizing Radiation,* Haley, T. J. and Snider, R., Eds., Academic Press, New York, 1962, 165.

314. Bateman, J. L. and Berdjis, C. C., Organs of special sense. I. Eye and irradiation, in *Pathology of Irradiation,* Berdjis, C. C., Ed., Williams & Wilkins, Baltimore, 1971, 669.

315. Berg, N. O. and Lindgren, M., Time-dose relationship and morphology of delayed radiation lesions of the brain in rabbits, *Acta Radiol. Suppl.,* 167, 1, 1958.

316. Boden, G., Radiation myelitis of the cervical spinal cord, *Br. J. Radiol.,* 21, 464, 1948.

317. Bogumill, G. P., Tissue changes in the brains of cats and monkeys following cobalt 60 irradiation, *Neurology,* 7, 245, 1957.

318. Bradley, E. W., Zook, B. C., Casarett, G. W., Bondelid, R. O., Maier, J. G., and Rogers, C. C., Effects of fast neutrons on rabbits. I. Comparison of pathologic effects of fractionated neutron and photon exposures of the head, *Int. J. Radiat. Oncol. Biol. Phys.,* 2, 1133, 1977.

319. Bradley, E. W., Zook, B. C., Casarett, G. W., Mossman, K. L., and Rogers, C. C., Effects of fast neutrons on rabbits. II. Comparison of pathologic effects of fractionated neutron and photon exposures of the lung and spinal cord, *Int. J. Radiat. Oncol. Biol. Phys.,* 5, 795, 1979.

320. Caveness, W. F., Roizin, L., Innes, J. R. M., and Carsten, A., Delayed effects of X-irradiation on the central nervous system of the monkey, in *Response of the Nervous System to Ionizing Radiation,* Haley, T. G. and Snider, R., Eds., Little, Brown, Boston, 1964.

321. Cogan, D. G., Ocular effects of radiation, *N. Engl. J. Med.,* 259, 517, 1958.

322. Dugger, G. S., Stratford, J. G., and Bouchard, J., Necrosis of the brain following roentgen irradiation, *Am. J. Roentgenol.,* 72, 953, 1954.

323. Dynes, J. B. and Smedal, M. I., Radiation myelitis, *Am. J. Roentgenol.,* 83, 78, 1960.

324. Evans, T. C., Richards, R. D., and Riley, E. F., Histologic studies of neutron- and X-irradiated mouse lenses, *Radiat. Res.,* 13, 737, 1960.

325. Gilmore, S. A., The effects of X-irradiation on the spinal cords of neonatal rats. II. Histological observations, *J. Neuropathol. Exp. Neurol.,* 22, 294, 1963.

326. Greenfield, M. M. and Stark, F. M., Post-irradiation neuropathology. *Am. J. Roentgenol.,* 60, 617, 1948.

327. Haley, T. J. and Snider, R., Eds., *Response of the Nervous System to Ionizing Radiation,* Academic Press, New York, 1962.

328. Haley, T. J. and Snider, R. S., Eds., *Response of the Nervous System to Ionizing Radiation,* Little, Brown, Boston, 1964.

329. Hanna, C. and O'Brien, J. E., Lens epithelial cell proliferation and migration in radiation cataracts, *Radiat. Res.,* 19, 1, 1963.

330. Haymaker, W., Effects of ionizing radiation on nervous tissue, in *Structure and Function of the Nervous System,* Vol. 3, Bourne, J., Ed., Academic Press, New York, 1969, chap., 10.

331. Innes, J. R. M. and Carsten, A., Delayed effects of localized X-irradiation of the nervous system of experimental rats and monkeys, in *Fundamental Aspects of Radiosensitivity,* Brookhaven National Laboratory Symposium in Biology, No. 14, 1961, 200.

332. Innes, J. R. M. and Carsten, A., in *Response of the Nervous System to Ionizing Radiation,* Haley, T. J. and Snider, R. S., Eds., Academic Press, New York, 1962, 233.

333. Jones, A., Transient radiation myelopathy (with reference to Lhermitte's sign of electrical paraesthesia), *Br. J. Radiol.,* 37, 727, 1964.

334. Kagan, E. H., Brownson, R. H., and Suter, D. B., Radiation-caused cytochemical changes in neurons, *Arch. Pathol.,* 74, 195, 1962.

335. Lampert, P., Tom, M. I., and Rider, W. D., Disseminated demyelination of the brain following $Co^{60}$ (gamma) radiation, *Arch. Pathol.,* 68, 322, 1959.

336. Larsson, B., Blood vessel changes following local irradiation of the brain with high energy protons, *Acta Soc. Med. Ups.,* 65, 61, 1960.

337. **Lerman, S.**, Radiation cataractogenesis, *N. Y. Med. J.*, 62, 3075, 1962.

338. **McDonald, L. W. and Hayes, T. L.**, The role of capillaries in the pathogenesis of delayed radionecrosis of brain, *Am. J. Pathol.*, 50, 745, 1967.

339. **McLaurin, R. L., Bailey, O. T., Harsh, G. R., and Ingraham, F. D.**, The effects of gamma and roentgen radiation on the intact spinal cord of the monkey, *Am. J. Roentgenol.*, 73, 827, 1955.

340. **Merriam, G. R., Jr., and Focht, E. F.**, A clinical study of radiation cataracts and the relationship to dose, *Am. J. Roentgenol.*, 77, 759, 1957.

341. **Merriam, G. R., Jr. and Focht, E. F.**, Radiation dose to the lens in treatment of tumors of the eye and adjacent structures. Possibilities of cataract formation, *Radiology*, 71, 357, 1958.

342. **Pallis, C. A., Louis, S. and Morgan, R. L.**, Radiation myelopathy, *Brain*, 84, 460, 1961.

343. **Pitcock, J. A.**, Demyelinating lesions and focal vascular lesions in the cerebral white matter of normal and irradiated monkeys (Macaca mulatta), *J. Neuropath. Exp. Neurol.*, 22, 120, 1963.

344. **Rider, W. D.**, Radiation damage to the brain — a new syndrome, *J. Can. Assoc. Radiol.*, 14, 67, 1963.

345. **Rogers, C. C., Bradley, E. W., Casarett, G.W., and Zook, B. C.**, Radiation myelopathy in dogs irradiated with fractionated fast neutrons or photons, *Radiat. Res.*, 74, 513, 1978.

346. **Von Sallmann, L., Tobias, C. A., Anger, H. O., Welch, C., Kimura, S. M., Munoz, C. M., and Drungis, A.**, Effects of high-energy particles, X-rays, and aging on lens epithelium, *Arch. Ophthalmol.*, 54, 489, 1955.

347. **Wanko, T., von Sallmann, L., and Gavin, M. A.**, Early changes in the lens epithelium after roentgen irradiation. A correlated light and electron microscopic study, *Arch. Ophthalmol.*, 62, 977, 1088, 1959.

348. **Warren, S.**, Effects on the nervous system. Effects of radiation on normal tissue, *Arch. Pathol.*, 35, 127, 1943.

349. **Zeman, W. and Solomon, M.**, Effects of irradiation on the nervous system, in *Pathology of Irradiation*, Berdjis, C. C., Ed., Williams & Wilkins, Baltimore, 1971, 213.

350. **Zook, B. C., Bradley, E. W., Casarett, G. W., and Rogers, C. C.**, Pathological anatomy of canine brain irradiated with fractionated fast neutrons or photons, *Radiat. Res.*, 74, 512, 1978.

351. **Andrews, G. A.**, Criticality accidents in Vinca, Jugoslvaia and Oak Ridge, Tennessee, *J.A.M.A.*, 179, 191, 1962.

352. **Bond, V. P.**, The role of infection in illness following exposure to acute total body irradiation, *Bull., N. Y. Acad. Med.*, 33, 369, 1957.

353. **Bond, V. P., Fliedner, T. M., and Cronkite, E. P.**, Evaluation and management of the heavily irradiated individual, *J. Nucl. Med.*, 1, 221, 1960.

354. **Casarett, G. W.**, Acceleration of aging by ionizing radiation, *J. Gerontol.*, 11, 436, 1956.

355. **Casarett, G. W.**, Acceleration of Aging by Ionizing Radiation, U.S. Atomic Energy Commission Report UR-492, Washington, D.C., 1957.

356. **Casarett, G. W.**, Acceleration of aging by ionizing radiations, in *Biological Aspects of Aging*, Strehler, B., Ed., Am. Inst. Biol. Sci., Washington, D. C., 1960, 147.

357. **Casarett, G. W.**, Radiologic aging, generalized and localized (with special reference to internal irradiation), in *Some Aspects of Internal Irradiation*, Dougherty, T. F. et al., Eds., Pergamon Press, New York, 1962, 251.

358. **Casarett, G. W.**, Possible effects of relatively low levels of radiation, *Monograph in Current Problems in Radiology*, Vol. III, No. 2, Year Book Medical Publishers, Chicago, 1973.

359. **Cronkite, E. P.**, The diagnosis, prognosis, and treatment of radiation injuries produced by atomic bombs, *Radiology*, 56, 661, 1951.

360. **Cronkite, E. P. and Bond, V. P.**, *Radiation Injury in Man, its Chemical and Biological Basis, Pathogenesis and Therapy*, Charles C Thomas, Springfield, Ill., 1960.

361. **Gerstner, H. B.**, Acute clinical effects of penetrating nuclear radiation, *J.A.M.A.*, 168, 381, 1958.

362. **Hempelmann, L. H., Lisco, H., and Hoffman, J. G.**, The acute radiation syndrome: a study of nine cases and a review of the problem, *Ann. Intern. Med.*, 36, 279, 1952.

363. **Ingram, M., Howland, J. W., and Hansen, C. H.**, Sequential manifestations of acute radiation injury vs. "acute radiation syndrome" stereotype, *Ann. N. Y. Acad. Sci.*, 114, 356, 1964.

364. International Atomic Energy Agency, *Diagnosis and Treatment of Acute Radiation Injury*, I.A.E.A., Vienna, 1961.

365. **Liebow, A. A., Warren, Ṡ., and De Coursey, E.**, Pathology of atomic bomb casualties, *Am. J. Pathol.*, 25, 853, 1949.

366. **Mathe, G., Amiel, J. L., and Schwarzenberg, L.**, Treatment of acute total-body irradiation injury in man, *Ann. N. Y. Acad. Sci.*, 114, 368, 1964.

367. National Academy of Sciences - National Research Council, *Treatment of Radiation Injury*, NAS-NRC Publication 134, Washington, D.C., 1964.

368. **Oughterson, A. W. and Warren, S.,** *Medical Effects of the Atomic Bomb in Japan,* McGraw-Hill, New York, 1956.

369. **Saenger, E. L.,** Medical Aspects of Radiation Accidents, U.S. Atomic Energy Commission, Washington, D.C., 1963.

370. **Thoma, G. E., Jr. and Wald, N.,** The diagnosis and management of the heavily irradiated individual, *J. Nucl. Med.,* 1, 421, 1959.

371. **Upton, A. C.,** The pathogenesis of the hemorrhagic state in radiation sickness, *Blood,* 10, 1156, 1955.

372. **Warren, S. and Bowers, J. Z.,** The acute radiation syndrome in man, *Ann. Intern. Med.,* 32, 207, 1950.

# INDEX